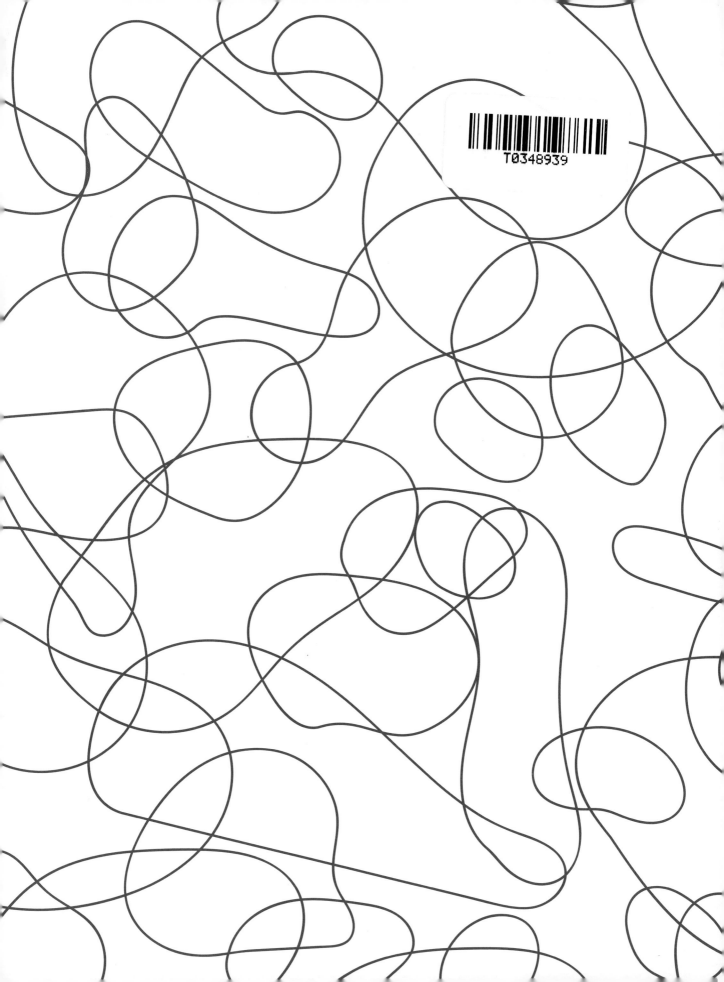

MENOPAUSE
MAKES

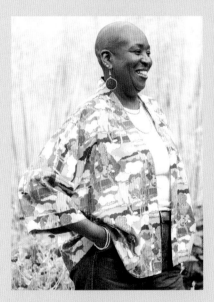
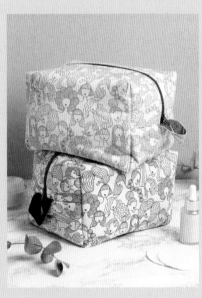
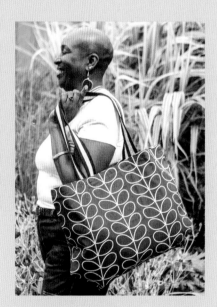

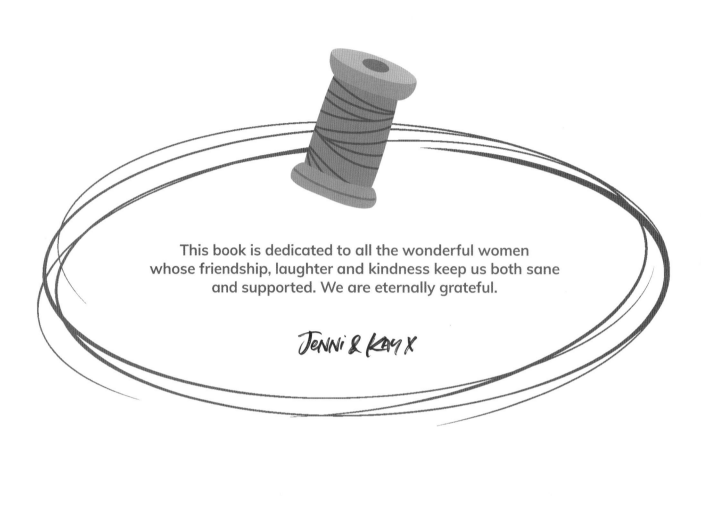

This book is dedicated to all the wonderful women
whose friendship, laughter and kindness keep us both sane
and supported. We are eternally grateful.

Jenni & Kay X

JENNI SMITH & KAY WALSH

MENOPAUSE MAKES

*EMPOWERING
SEWING PROJECTS
TO RELAX YOUR MIND,
COOL YOUR BODY
AND IGNITE
YOUR CREATIVITY*

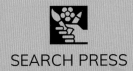

SEARCH PRESS

CONTENTS

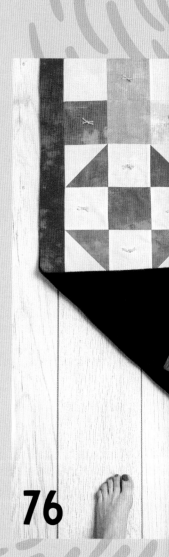

6   What is the menopause?
FOREWORD BY DR HANNAH DAVIES

10   Welcome to Menopause Makes

16   Materials & tools

26   Choosing colours

28   How to use this book

30   THE PROJECTS

    32   INSOMNIA: SLEEP MASK
       38   GUEST DESIGNER SALLY KELLY

    40   MEMORY LOSS: BASKET FOR LOST THINGS
       46   GUEST DESIGNER KAREN LEWIS

    48   LOW MOOD: WEEKEND-AWAY TOTE

    54   DRY, ITCHY SKIN: ZIPPED POTION POUCH
       62   GUEST DESIGNER RASHIDA COLEMAN-HALE

    64   STRESS: LOG CABIN PLACEMATS

    70   BRAIN FOG: FLYING GEESE PILLOW

    76   ANXIETY: RELAXATION BLANKET

    86   BUTTER FINGERS: MAKER'S APRON

    94   HOT FLASHES: COOL-DOWN COVER-UP
       104   GUEST DESIGNER ALICE GARRETT

    106   NIGHT SWEATS: KEEP COOL QUILT

120   Tips & techniques

146   Resources

147   Thanks & acknowledgements

148   Glossary

150   Index

76

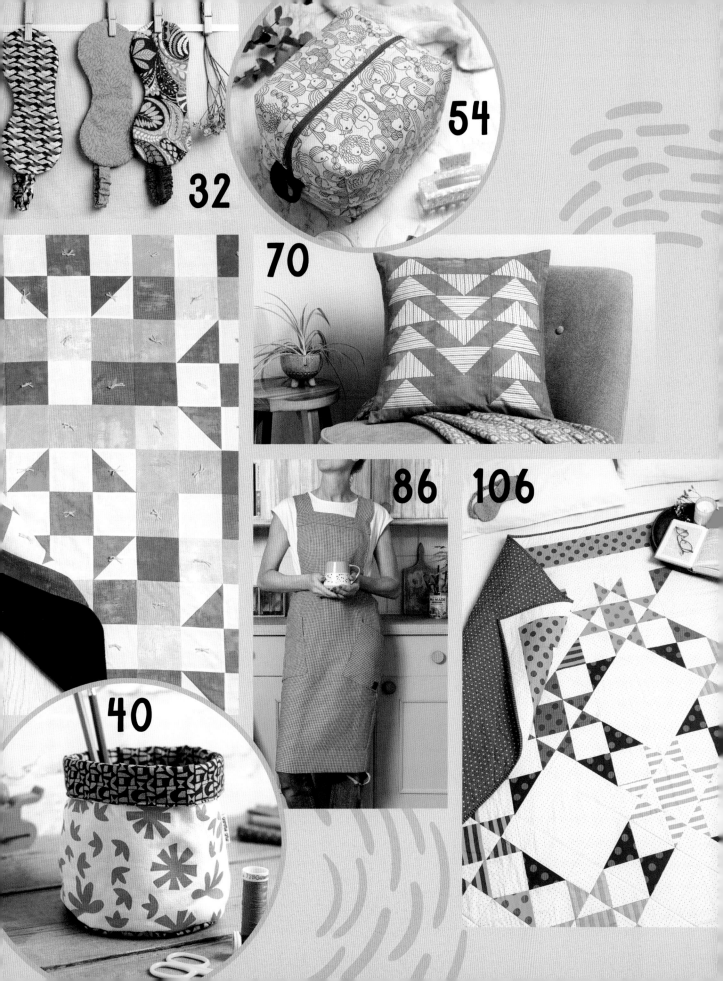

32

54

70

86 106

40

WHAT IS THE MENOPAUSE?

Foreword by Dr Hannah Davies

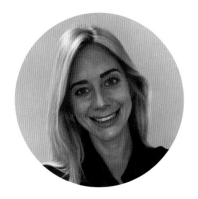

Hannah Davies (BSc MBBS MRCGP) is a doctor specializing in the menopause and lifestyle medicine. After obtaining a First Class degree in Biomedical Science at University College London, and earning a place on the Dean's List in recognition of her outstanding performance, she then went on to study Medicine at University College London, graduated in 2016, and became a fully qualified GP after a further 5 years of postgraduate training.

When Hannah began GP training, she quickly started to gain huge levels of satisfaction from providing high-quality, compassionate, patient-led menopause care to her patients, which has driven her to pursue a specialist interest in the menopause. She loves empowering women, and equipping them with the necessary knowledge and tools to make their own personalized, informed decisions about managing their menopause.

> *IT is time THAT THe MeNOPAUSe iS SeeN AS A ceLeBRATORY MiLeSTONe To Be eMBRACeD WiTHOUT PANiC AND SHAMe.*

Historically, menopause has been perceived as a negative consequence of aging, and associated with not only the demise of fertility but also femininity. In the early 1900s, the menopause was pathologized and framed as a severe deficiency disease affecting women at the end of their life. For a woman, it was a phase that was dreaded: menopausal women were vilified or dismissed, due to superstitions about an aging female body, and the propaganda proclaiming that women's biological and social purpose ended with menopause.

Although in recent times steps have been made to improve our understanding of this stage in a woman's life, the menopause remains under-researched (in parallel with all female hormonal health problems) and under-appreciated. This means this landmark period of every woman's life is still shrouded in myths and misunderstandings, which remain woven into the culture of trivialization and stigmatization today.

Female lifespan now far exceeds a woman's reproductive lifespan, meaning that most women will spend about 30–40% of their lives post-menopause. By 2030, 1 billion women across the world will have entered or will be about to enter menopause. These numbers alone should make a convincing argument to direct our attention towards a better understanding of the menopause, to not only improve the health of women worldwide but to change the current menopausal landscape to one that women can embrace, celebrate and thrive in.

The textbook definitions of menopause serve only to confine this period of a woman's life to their sexual function, and feed into the narrative that women are defined by their reproductive and sexual systems. The World Health Organization defines the menopause as the permanent end of menstruation (more commonly known as 'periods') due to a loss of ovarian follicular activity. However, this arbitrary definition fails to acknowledge that the significant hormonal changes that accompany the perimenopause and menopause impact every single organ in the body, and not just those confined to the pelvis. It manifests in an array of symptoms from the physical (hot flashes, night sweats, joint pains, palpitations, dizziness, and dryness of the eyes, mouth, skin, hair and vagina) to the psychological (irritability, rage, tearfulness and anxiety, as well as cognitive disturbance, which can be far more profound than the colloquial phrase 'brain fog' would lead many to believe).

Further still, these objective definitions fail to encompass the physiological processes that ensue as women enter the perimenopause. There's a decrease in bone mass, muscle mass and collagen, and increasing postprandial glucose, cholesterol, uric acid, visceral fat and blood pressure, which collectively place menopausal women at a greater risk of osteoporosis, type 2 diabetes, heart disease, dementia, cancer and stroke, than their pre-menopausal counterparts.

Such definitions also fail to acknowledge the psychosocial impact that the menopause can inflict on women's lives. An estimated 59% of women have taken time off work, 51% have reduced their working hours due to menopausal symptoms, and 73% of women report the menopause playing a role in their divorce.

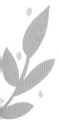

While the menopausal landscape is changing, the historical narrative of what it means to be 'menopausal' remains an unconscious bias that not only influences how women are perceived and treated by physicians, but arguably more importantly, how woman perceive themselves. It is time that the menopause is seen through a holistic lens that acknowledges the systemic impact that menopause inflicts upon the entirety of the female body, beyond the limitations of the ovaries and uterus. It is time that the menopause is seen as a celebratory milestone to be embraced without panic or shame, and it is time that menopausal women are encouraged to speak out and seek help in a culture that fosters understanding, acceptance and inclusive care around menopause.

Unhelpfully, the menopause is a diagnosis made in retrospect once a woman has missed 12 consecutive periods, and there are no accurate or precise biological tests to predict when this might happen. Consequently, symptoms of the perimenopause, which may begin up to 10 years before the menopause, often go misdiagnosed – too frequently as mental illness – or unrecognized, leaving women to suffer needlessly.

Women navigating the perimenopause may have a more challenging time than post-menopausal women, owing to the fact that their hormones (oestrogen and progesterone) are on a rollercoaster of a journey. While there is a general downward trajectory of ovarian hormone production, there will be many highs and lows along the way. During the perimenopause, a woman's oestrogen level may be at the highest it has ever been and then plummets to the lowest level, and it is this huge variation and instability in hormone levels that can give rise to the plethora of menopausal symptoms described above, alongside unpredictable changes to the menstrual cycle that range from incredibly heavy bleeding to scanty light periods, and anything in between.

Once post-menopausal (12 months after that last-ever period), the physical, emotional, and mental load often settles. While a post-menopausal woman has a very low oestrogen level – 1% of her former pre-menopausal self and in lower quantities than a man of the same age – the hormone levels plateau and stabilize. This tends to translate into a lower burden of symptoms for many women, and often leads to a period of life filled with contentment and greater life satisfaction.

In contrast to preconceived ideas and notions that menopausal marketing would have you believe, studies performed across the nations have shown that post-menopausal women are happier and more satisfied than they were in earlier pre-menopausal years. Such insights challenge the menopausal stereotype of a disgruntled, hot, old woman. It is important we lean into more positive studies and start looking at the menopause under a broader lens, which offers a new definition of the menopause, one which associates this period of profound hormonal change with new meaning and purpose. In fact, shifting one's mindset and contemplating the menopause as a chapter of your life associated with liberation and opportunity, may serve you well with respect to reducing your symptomatic burden. In those cultures where the menopause is welcomed as an important aging landmark, and is associated with higher societal status and a sense of achievement, women report significantly fewer menopausal symptoms.

While it would be cruel and unjust to suggest to any woman that their symptoms are the result of a negative mindset (because we know the very real biological upheavals that are at play), recognizing the power of the mind-body connection gives women back their autonomy and allows a sense of control over their menopausal journey. Using a holistic tool kit comprised of healthy-habit stacking – metacognition (being aware of your own thought processes and the reasons behind them), diet, movement and more – women can feel empowered as they begin this phase of life, all while seeing the menopause with a new enlightened perspective. For many women, hormone replacement therapy (HRT) will be part of this tool kit that helps them thrive during the menopause, and the effectiveness of HRT cannot be under-estimated. For other women, for individual reasons, HRT may not be their lifeline. No two women will have the same menopausal experience, and here within lies the nuance of the menopause. Therefore, it stands to reason that menopausal care and treatment is, and must be, unique to each woman.

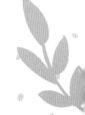

...THE ACTIVITY OF SEWING PROVIDES A BASIS FOR SOCIAL CONNECTION WITH OTHERS, WHICH IS WELL KNOWN TO IMPROVE MENTAL WELL-BEING.

I feel honoured to write the foreword for this innovative and imaginative book. Sewing, and craft in general, is gaining increasing popularity, no doubt in part due to media coverage of well-known celebrities and sporting heroes demonstrating their love for it. Perhaps more important, is the increasing awareness of the therapeutic benefits that can be derived from this long-appreciated pastime.

The average age for the menopause in the UK is 51. This time in life is often associated with significant social shifts, such as changing occupational status and changes in marital status, while simultaneously caring for children and elderly parents, and both coincide with an increased risk of health problems. This culminates in unprecedented levels of stress. Stress plays havoc on our hormonal health, and high stress levels will only heighten menopausal symptoms. Making something with your hands has long been known for its stress-relieving benefits and therefore, this book provides an invaluable tool for women in search of something which will tap into their parasympathetic nervous system, lower their cortisol (stress hormone) levels, and provide a moment of calm. Sewing has long been known to reduce anxiety, still the mind and, for some, provides a form of meditative practice, which has never been more needed than during those perimenopausal years.

Menopause is associated with a number of cerebral structural, metabolic and chemical changes, which increase the risk for cognitive decline, therefore optimizing brain health needs to be a top priority during this chapter of a woman's life. Learning a new skill, such as sewing, builds new neural connections and has been shown to improve cognitive and functional abilities. Through such cognitive stimulation you can help craft a more resilient brain that is more resistant to dementia, the incidence of which increases significantly post-menopause – yet another benefit to picking up, or continuing, this hobby in later life.

Further still, the activity of sewing provides a basis for social connection with others, which is well known to relieve stress and improve mental well-being. Social connections are associated with happier and healthier individuals who live longer than those who are socially isolated, and women with a stronger support system tend to exhibit greater resilience in response to menopausal symptoms, which alone makes the concept of a sewing community even more enticing.

The menopause is all part of life's rich tapestry. Whether you are nervous of this time or see it as a chance to curate a new healthy lifestyle enriched with new experiences is up to you, and more importantly, the tools you choose to help you along the way are personal and unique to you. Whichever you choose, it's yours to experience.

MAKING SOMETHING WITH YOUR HANDS HAS LONG BEEN KNOWN FOR ITS STRESS-RELIEVING BENEFITS... AN INVALUABLE TOOL FOR WOMEN.

WELCOME TO
MENOPAUSE MAKES

The mission of this book is to bring colour and creativity into the lives of women experiencing perimenopause and menopause; to build their skills and confidence in sewing, and to make projects that have the ability to positively impact their mood and daily lives.

Each project in this book provides a hand-made solution to a challenge faced during this massive hormonal shift, and is designed to be both functional and fun.

Together, we can make a foggy time feel clearer, and counter any feelings of loneliness and isolation by building a strong, creative community of 'Menopausal Makers' around the world.

What are we waiting for...?

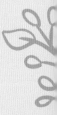

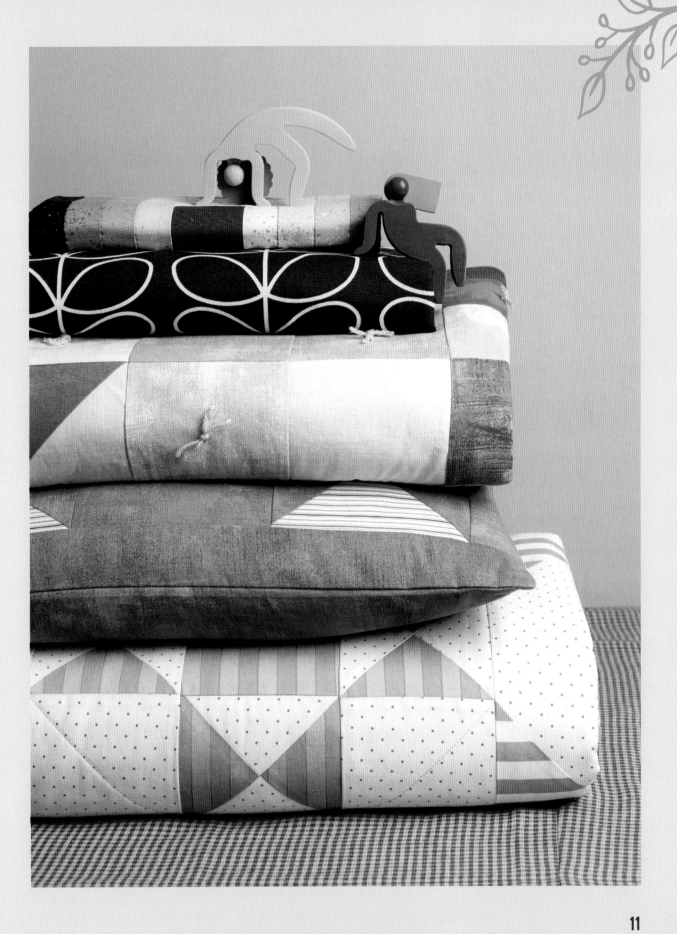

ABOUT US

TAP DANCING & TEARS

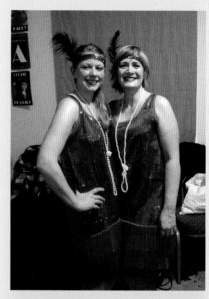

We're Jenni and Kay, globe-trotting quilting and dressmaking teachers, authors and makers based in Ilkley, West Yorkshire, UK, and we are on a mission to get everyone stitching and smiling!

We have been sewing for over 30 years, and we count ourselves fortunate that our love of stitching and quilting has been fuelled by our friendship and the rich textile history in the north of England.

We met in our mid-thirties at our local tap-dancing class. It wasn't long before I (Jenni) gently persuaded Kay to also get creative with a needle and thread, teaching her to quilt with a group of friends around the kitchen table (reliably accompanied by a constant flow of Yorkshire tea!).

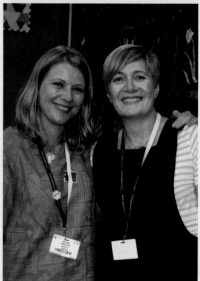

Soon most social gatherings inevitably involved stitching. As our friendship grew, so did our love of making our own clothes and clothes for the children, sewing decorations for our home, patchworking and stitching gifts. Much fabric was bought, and laughter was the soundtrack of those early experiments – making something with a little skill and a lot of enthusiasm!

Our crafty community grew into a bustling studio and was the catalyst for us to launch our own patterns, inspire community projects and author a book collaboration with Liberty™.

Most days are spent in each other's company, as well as with the many marvellous women we meet. While our hands are busy making, we take the time to process life's ups and downs with every stitch. Tears of laughter are still falling in the studio, but there are tears of sadness, anger and frustration too.

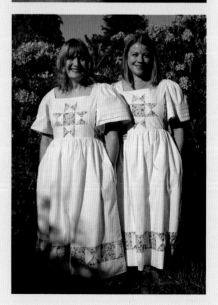

Sweet clothes for the kids are now farewell gifts as they fly the nest; fitted blouses are replaced by looser, stylish cover-ups; and cozy quilts need to be much lighter if there is any hope of sleeping beneath them! The same skills are in use, but for different reasons.

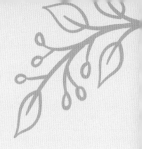

OUR MENOPAUSE EXPERIENCE

As I (Kay) hit my mid-forties, I began to notice huge changes to both my body and mind, often leaving me feeling tired, angry and sad. As an avid reader and listener of podcasts, discussions around perimenopause piqued my curiosity, and I armed myself with as much knowledge as possible before visiting my GP. Despite this, it still took resilience and numerous visits before being prescribed HRT, and the past eight years have been a journey of shifting perspectives to really look after myself (though I am still often way too hot!). I find it disheartening that many friends in the same position are still being offered anti-depressants, or encouraged to 'battle on', without any alternative solutions.

For me (Jenni), having Kay a few years older and already on her 'menopause mission' is a real life-saver. A couple of years ago, I became noticeably more anxious, which for me as a pretty laid-back person was very unnerving and quite a shock. It is surprisingly easy to put up with 'not quite feeling like yourself', and accepting light-hearted criticism from others about your mood swings, but the struggle is real. Staying informed and strong are essential tools for surviving this hormonal shift, and again HRT, exercise and creativity have landed me in a much happier place (although I can't always remember where that place is due to the brain fog!).

Luckily for us, we have each other and stitching to help us along this journey.

WHY WE ARE PROUD OF THIS BOOK!

Menopause Makes was born from our genuine desire to empower women at a time when their mental health, self-esteem and well-being can suffer.

Our hope is to extend the support we've felt to other women, and make manageable projects that inspire pride and positivity. We truly believe the magic of sewing is that it really can help you slow down enough to at least acknowledge the present moment and then plan how to take your next step forward – one stitch at a time.

We're also thrilled to spotlight four amazing designers across the world who share our passion for a 'creative menopause'. In no particular order, we'd like to introduce Sally Kelly, Rashida Coleman-Hale, Karen Lewis and Alice Garrett. We're delighted to be using and featuring a selection of designs from their gorgeous fabric collections in this book.

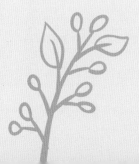

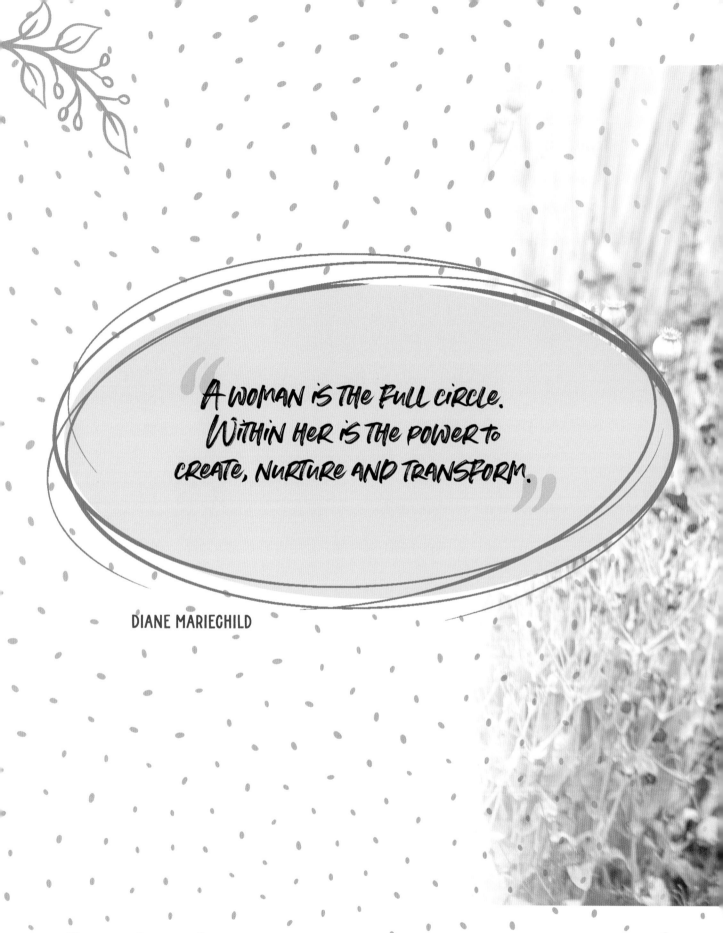

"A woman is the full circle.
Within her is the power to
create, nurture and transform."

DIANE MARIECHILD

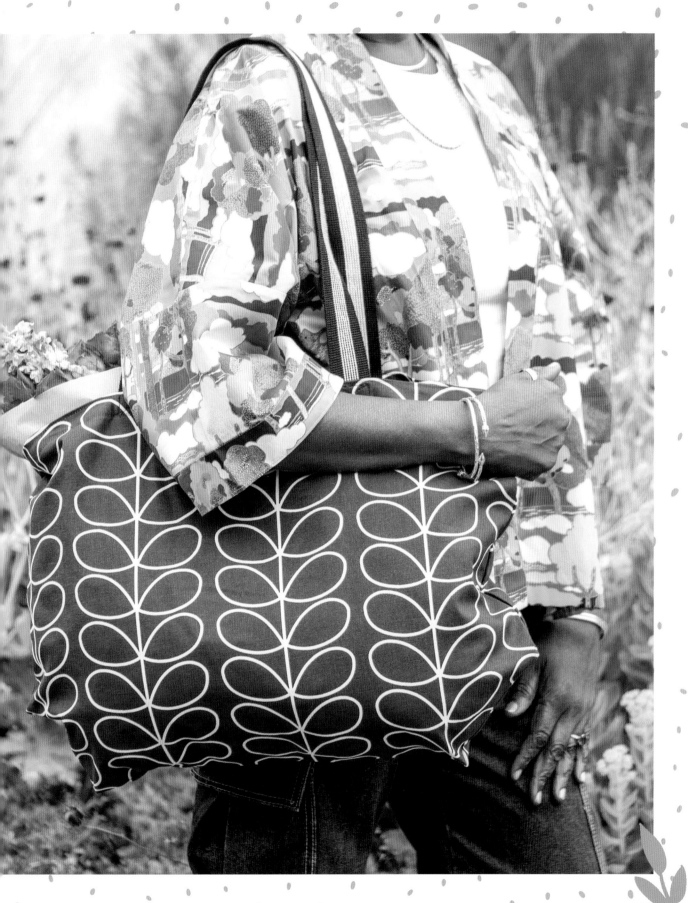

MATERIALS
& TOOLS

Here is a user-friendly guide to suggested tools you'll need for your *Menopause Makes* projects, all of which we have tried and tested over many years of sewing.

We've also included some advice on the different fabrics you can use, to ensure you get the finish you love.

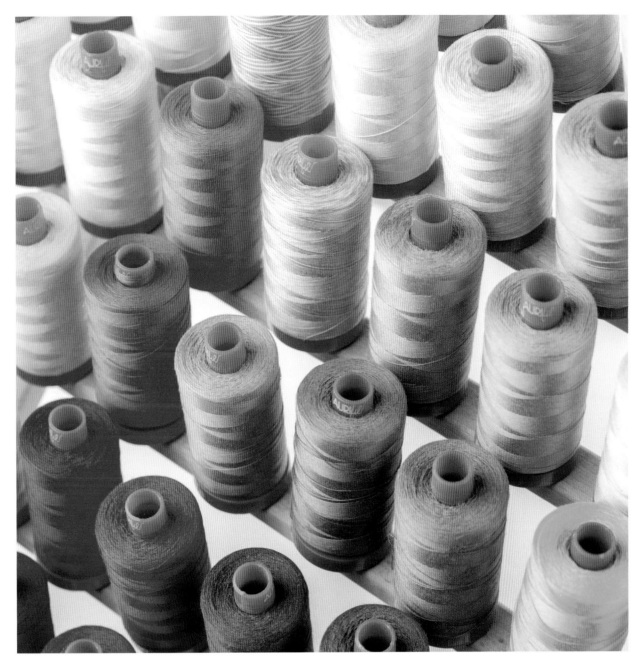

MATERIALS

THREAD

Always choose a good-quality thread – cheap ones snap easily and can cause real frustration. We recommend 100% cotton, especially for the patchwork projects: it creates flat seams, and doesn't harm your fabric if it needs to be unpicked. Aurifil is our favourite brand to use, as it is lint-free (meaning no fluff in your sewing machine!), and comes in different weights and stunning colours. More details on the most suitable weight is given where necessary.

FABRICS

We have designed the 10 projects in this book to give you the perfect opportunity to use different fabrics, and extend your knowledge on how they behave. Sometimes, stepping beyond what feels like the safest option can bring stunning results.

So, what are your choices?

COTTON

- 100% cotton is very versatile and available in so many beautiful colours and printed designs. It features a lot in this book!

- Quilting cotton is generally slightly heavier than dressmaking cotton, but they can be interchangeable and also used together in one project.

- Don't be tempted to use a cotton/polyester blend, especially when piecing patchwork. This alternative can be more cost effective, but can distort easily and might leave you disappointed with the finished result.

COTTON LAWN

- This variation of cotton has a finer weave than quilting or dressmaking cotton, and feels more like silk. However, it is easier to handle than silk and has a floaty, light-weight quality, making it perfect for the Cool-down Cover-up (see page 94).

- It is suitable for use in patchwork projects and can be used alongside quilting cotton if you desire.

- The most famous brand of cotton lawn is Tana Lawn™ by Liberty™ – and it is a firm favourite in our studio!

SILK

- Like cotton, silk is a natural fibre. The trickiest part of handling silk is cutting it out. If possible, cut it with a rotary cutter, cutting mat and pattern weights to avoid it slipping out of position. Also choose fine pins, needles and cotton thread when sewing with it.

LINEN

- This natural fibre is strong, durable and doesn't stain easily. It absorbs moisture and adapts well to different temperatures. For these reasons, it is the perfect choice for garments – especially aprons, such as our Maker's Apron (see page 86), which get a lot of wear.

- Linen frays more than cotton, but sewing with French seams (see pages 89 and 98) can keep this under control.

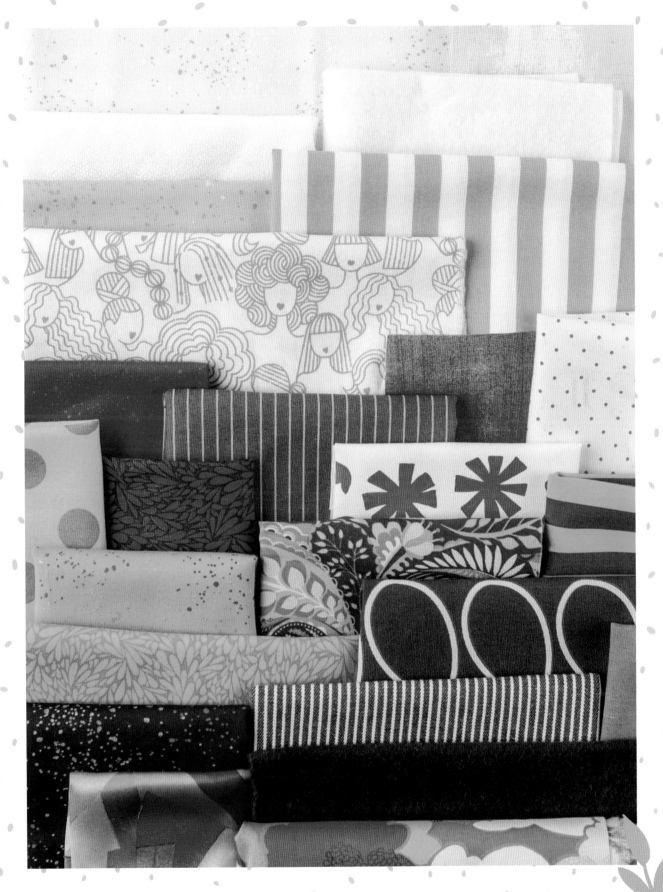

FURNISHING/UPHOLSTERY FABRIC

- This is a heavy-weight 100% cotton fabric that lends itself to bags – such as our Weekend-away Tote (see page 48) – due to its strength and ability to provide structure.

- Denim is often a similar weight and would make a good alternative.

- Furnishing fabric is not ideal for patchwork as it is harder to get precise points with heavier weight fabrics.

FLEECE

- There are many types of fleece available but we would only recommend one which is made of 100% cotton (and is organic, if possible). It is soft and cozy (and wide) so great to use as backing fabric for a blanket or throw – like our Relaxation Blanket (see page 76).

BATTING/WADDING

This fabric is the middle layer of a traditional quilt, adding padding, warmth and depth.

It comes in many different variations including 100% cotton, wool, polyester and bamboo. The most common (and the one we would recommend for the Keep Cool Quilt on page 106) is an 80/20 blend, i.e. 80% cotton and 20% polyester. It can be purchased off the bolt by the yard or metre, or in pre-cut packs depending on the size you require, for example King Size, Crib Size, and so on.

If you want a super-light quilt, you could try bamboo as this is thin yet strong and has a lovely drape. However, typically it is more expensive than a cotton blend.

Should I prewash my fabric?

We do, and if you choose to do so, you should do this before you cut into your fabric, in case of shrinkage. Generally, shrinkage is minimal and usually less than 5%, so in patchwork you may not even notice. However, in dressmaking it could affect the final fit of your garment. Before cutting out, press the fabric after washing to ensure there are no wrinkles and there's no distortion.

"Act as young as you feel. You're not getting older, you're getting more entitled to be your fabulous self."

GWEN STEFANI

TOOLS

SEWING MACHINE

All the projects are manageable on a standard sewing machine, even the larger Relaxation Blanket (see page 76) and Keep Cool Quilt (see page 106). If you haven't used your machine for a while, give it a dust, ensure that you clean out the bobbin holder and install a new machine needle.

If you need guidance on setting up your machine, always refer to the manual that comes with it; every machine is different, so although there will be similar features across some machines, it's worth familiarizing yourself with the ones specific to your model.

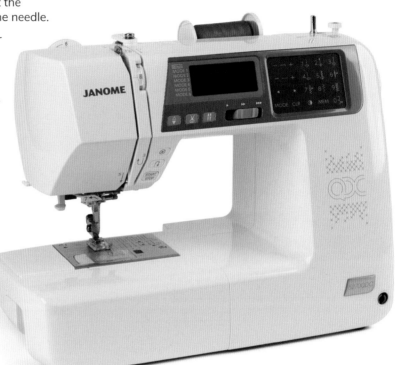

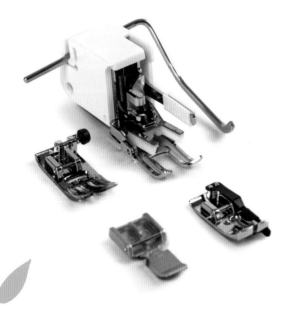

SEWING-MACHINE FEET

Alongside the standard foot that comes with your machine, you need a walking (even-/dual-feed) foot for any quilting; a zipper foot for the Zipped Potion Pouch (see page 54); and a ¼in foot for sewing together patchwork pieces (known as 'piecing') for the Flying Geese Pillow (see page 70), Relaxation Blanket (see page 76) and the Keep Cool Quilt (see page 106). The regular foot, zipper foot and ¼in foot can all be attached to the standard foot holder on your machine. Note that the walking foot may be a separate attachment that needs to be screwed into position; refer to your sewing machine manual for detailed instructions if this is the case.

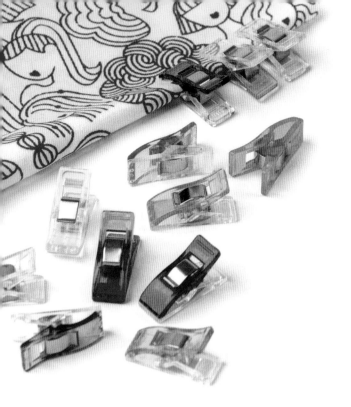

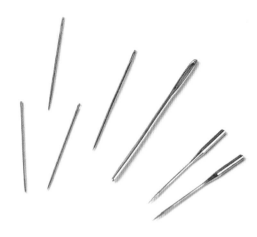

NEEDLES

Choose the appropriate machine needle for the project and the fabric it needs to stitch through. Needle size is also determined by the thread, which needs to fit through the eye of the needle. So, finding ones that work well together is essential.

For most projects we recommend a universal needle in size 80/12 which is great for sewing cotton fabrics. For heavier fabrics you should use a 90/14 needle and a heavier thread.

If you can hear a popping sound when your machine is sewing, generally it means that your needle is struggling. Taking a little time to get this part of your set-up correct can make a big difference to the overall quality of the project. More details are given in the materials list of each project. After use, why not attach your needle onto a piece of the fabric it works for as a quick reference next time you need it; this is much easier than trying to read the tiny size stamps on them!

For hand quilting, we like to use:

- 50wt or 40wt thread with John James Sharps or quilting needles in size 10

- 12wt thread with John James Embroidery needles in size 3 or 5.

For machine quilting, we like to use:

- 50wt or 40wt thread with an 80/12 needle

- 28wt thread with a 90/14 needle.

PINS

Fine, sharp pins are important if you don't want to snag your fabric. Glass-headed ones don't melt if they get close to an iron so they are always a favourite. Please don't use ones that have been lying around for years and are rusted – treat yourself to a new box! You may also find a magnetic pincushion extremely useful for sweeping up dropped pins at the end of the day.

SEWING/FABRIC CLIPS

These are a popular alternative to pins, especially if you're working with bulky projects. They are life-savers for the Basket for Lost Things (see page 40), the Weekend-away Tote (see page 48) and the Maker's Apron (see page 86).

SEAM RIPPER/QUICK UNPICK

Sewing machines may come with a free seam ripper but we prefer to purchase one that has an ergonomic handle – ideal if it is going to get lots of use!

SCISSORS

It is super important to choose a pair of scissors that feels comfortable in your hand, with blades that are sharp enough to cut right to the tips, so be careful not to go for style over substance. It is useful to have a mix of scissors: dressmaking shears, smaller embroidery scissors, and craft scissors only used for paper.

ROTARY CUTTER & CUTTING MAT

A rotary cutter is an alternative to scissors when cutting out fabrics, especially patchwork. It can cause less strain, you can go through multiple layers of fabric and it saves time. Our favourite is an Olfa with a 45mm replaceable blade.

Self-healing mats are used together with a rotary cutter. Choose a size which is workable in your sewing space, and has imperial (inch) measurements and degree markings on it. The most usable size of mat for the projects in this book would be around 36 x 24in (or A1/90 x 60cm) size, and it can always be stored away easily beneath furniture when not in use.

MEASURING TOOLS

We use two kinds: a tape measure and quilt rulers.

Tape measures are useful for lots of sewing projects. It's not recommended to use tape measures made of fabric, as these can stretch with use, so stick to ones made of plastic.

Quilting rulers are essential for patchwork. When choosing ones to buy, our main criteria is clear visibility of the ¼in markings. The ideal duo when starting out is one large 6 x 24in (15.25 x 61cm) ruler and a 6½in (16.5cm) square.

POINT TURNER

Poking scissors into the corner of a project will never end well, so we recommend using a chopstick. If you get into sewing, you can buy point turners relatively cheaply. They can be made of plastic or you can buy very nice bamboo or wooden ones.

PRESSING CLOTH

This is a cheap and extremely useful item to have when sewing projects, especially if you're working with garments and fabric that need to have interfacing applied. Choose white or unbleached cotton muslin (½yd or 50cm is plenty) and cut it into multiple pieces that are approximately the same dimensions as a tea towel. Simply place the pressing cloth between your fabric and the iron, then press as normal. Use it damp if you want to generate some steam.

SEAM GAUGE

This is an inexpensive metal measuring tool that's very useful when marking seams in dressmaking. It's also handy to use alongside the iron when pressing, as it doesn't melt like a regular tape measure!

COLOUR CATCHERS

These are always worth having when you wash a finished project for the first time, especially patchwork projects where multiple fabrics are used.

BASTING/TACKING TOOLS

There are different options when temporarily joining the layers of a quilt or blanket before stitching. Odif 505 basting spray is very effective, or you can use curved safety pins (which are easier to slide through multiple layers of fabric than straight versions).

MARKING TOOLS

There are multiple tools that can be used for marking out your quilt lines, such as the ones listed below. Always test your preferred marking tool on a scrap of fabric first.

- Water-soluble fabric marker pen – the ink for these will come out when the quilt is washed.
- Fabric pencil or chalk pencil – the marks of both can either be erased or washed out.
- Hera marker, which is a plastic or bamboo tool with a sharp edge that leaves a visible crease line on the quilt top that you can then follow. It should be used along with a quilting ruler to mark the lines.

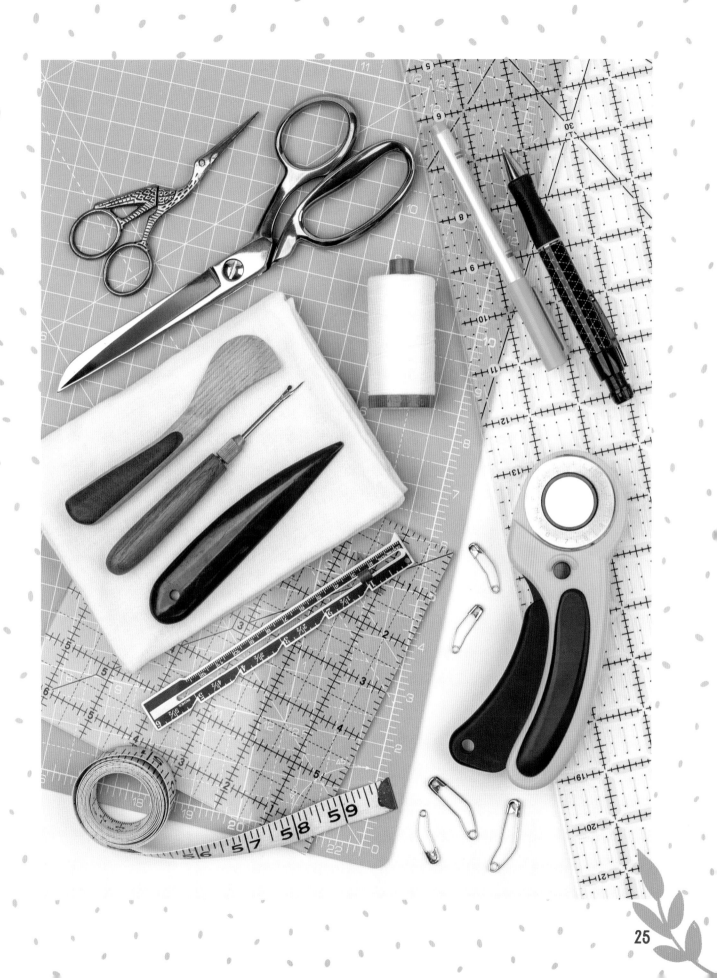

CHOOSING
COLOURS

Having taught hundreds of students over the years, we know that choosing fabric colours and feeling confident about whether they work or not is hard, and may even stop a project before you've even started.

We could spend the next few pages diving into colour theory and studying colour wheels, but we have also learned that trusting your own instinct and taste has enormous value! You are a woman with a good number of years of experience at choosing clothes to wear, styling interiors and soaking up culture, so why not try one or all of our four colour-confidence builders, opposite, as the launch pad for your *Menopause Makes* projects.

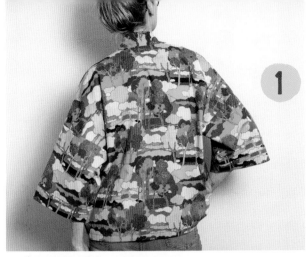

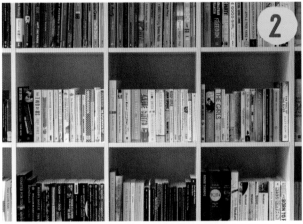

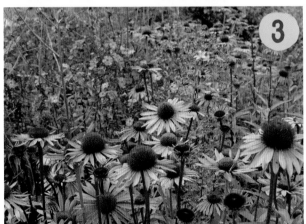

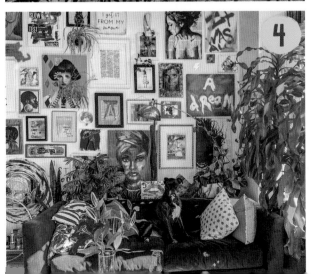

- **Select your favourite item of clothing or outfit in your wardrobe and use the colours as your palette (1).** If everything is one colour, think how you might accessorize your clothing with shoes, handbags and jewellery, and what colours they would be. Are your clothes predominately printed designs or solids? This can also influence the kind of fabrics you choose. And don't think that a solid colour means a project is boring – a single, plain shade can be very striking.

- **Leaf through your bookshelf (2) and select a book you were drawn to because you loved the cover and the design selections made by its illustrator.** Pick out the key colours and use those in your project. You could do the same with an album cover, painting or fabric design. Take a peek at the Liberty™ print Prospect Road fabric we've used for the Cool-down Cover-up (see the top image on this page, and page 94), which was the inspiration for the book's colour palette.

- **Let nature be your teacher (3)!** Don't overlook the world that surrounds you and the striking colour combinations that can be found in the countryside, in a flower bed, or on the feathers of your favourite bird. Pick a scene, and either in person or via a photograph note the colours that really sing together for you.

- A lot of your personality goes into decorating your home and choosing soft furnishings, and these choices will most likely bring you comfort because they're familiar and you're surrounded by them each day. **Use your home design as a spring board (4)** for a project's colour thinking especially about which shades and patterns dominate, and what pops of colour you can introduce to keep the eye moving.

HOW TO USE THIS
BOOK

All the projects in this book are achievable, even if you are a beginner, and have been designed with many of the common symptoms of menopause in mind. Tune in to your body and mind to help pick the project that works for you at a particular time.

Each of our 10 *Menopause Makes* projects starts with a description of the symptom that it relates to, and how it can help; use this as a guide to get started. For example, if insomnia is creeping in, the Sleep Mask will prove invaluable.

Getting started is often the biggest hurdle, but many of the projects in this book can be completed in just a few hours. Quilts and garments require bigger investments of time but are equally very rewarding, so we suggest picking a project that you connect with and enjoy the journey of stitching it, without putting pressure on yourself to reach the finish line. Nothing beats the feeling of saying 'I made this myself!'

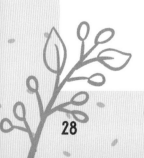

1 Difficulty rating: Every project has been rated with one of the three following skill levels:

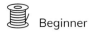 Beginner

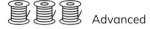 Intermediate

🧵🧵🧵 Advanced

If you're new to sewing, we recommend strongly that you start with the beginner projects, then work your way upwards.

2 Finished size: The final dimensions of a project, once it's made.

3 Notes: Here, we've detailed the seam allowance we've used for the project (which will vary from project to project), as well as any special techniques or useful extra information to be aware of before starting.

4 You will need: On top of the equipment detailed on pages 16–25, this is a list of everything you'll need for this particular project.

5 Cutting instructions: In addition to an overall requirements list, we've provided details on what you need to cut out before making up your projects. Lots of patterns do this, so you can get the more boring cutting-out bit done in one go, and then get on with the much more exciting stage: sewing!

6 Photographs: Every project is accompanied by pictures of our own version of it, not only to provide inspiration but also to give you extra visual information about its features. Sometimes we've made the item more than once, so you can see what it looks like in alternative fabrics too.

7 Method: This is where you find out how to make your project. We've broken down the instructions into steps, with illustrations of key stages to give you helpful, visual guidance.

8 Tip boxes: If there is something to bear in mind when making your project, or an extra tip, we'll pop it in a tip box for added support.

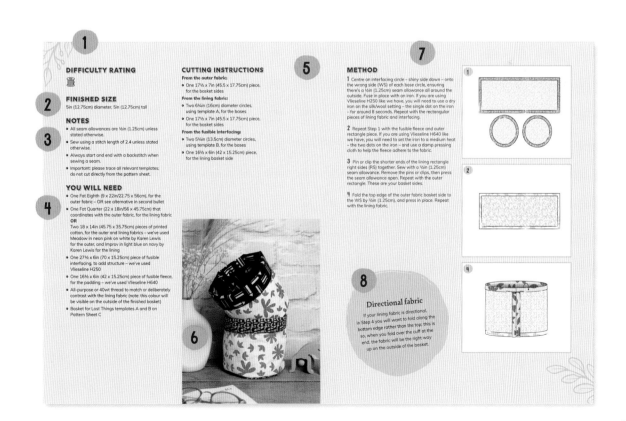

The PROJECTS

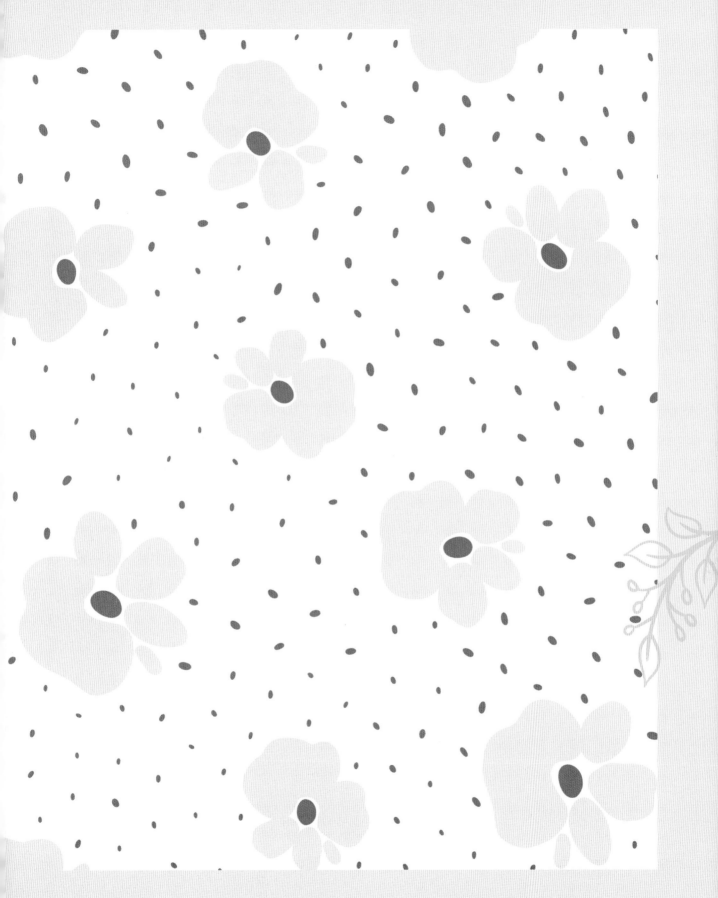

Symptom #1

INSOMNIA

During menopause, sleep is often disrupted, anxious, hot, and in too-short supply. Wearing a sleep mask is one constructive step to improving the chance of a proper night's rest. Block out unwanted light (or attention!) and make it part of a bedtime routine that is focused on truly switching off. You can't scroll on your phone when your eyes are covered!

This project is the perfect way to kick-start your sewing journey because it is not only simple to construct, but practical too. The small fabric requirements also means this sleep mask is cost-effective to sew, and it would make a great last-minute gift for a sleep-deprived girlfriend.

We've deliberately made the mask reversible, in case you'd like to use more than one print for it. Have fun choosing the prints – however outlandish they may be – as they are only seen in the bedroom!

SLEEP MASK

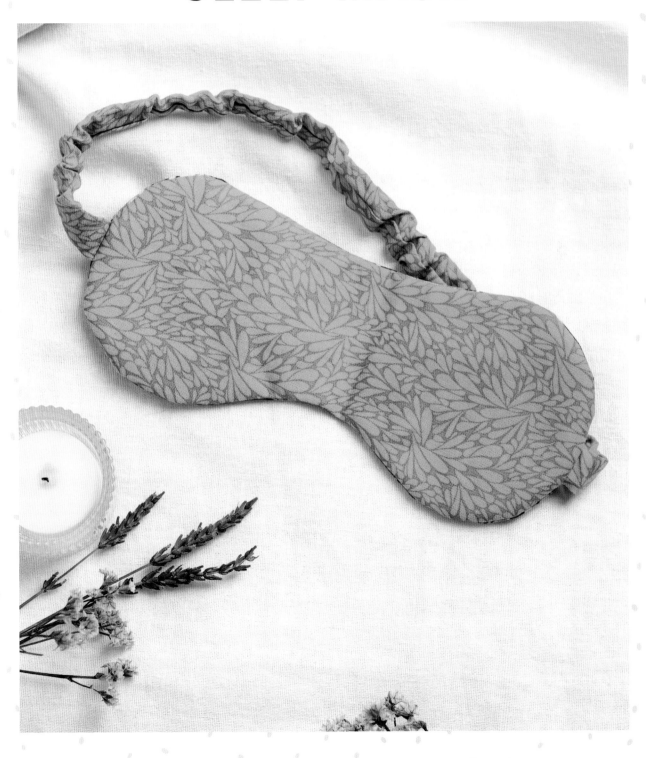

DIFFICULTY RATING

FINISHED SIZE

8 x 3in (20.25 x 7.5cm)

NOTES

- All seam allowances are ⅜in (1cm) unless stated otherwise.
- Sew using a stitch length of 2.4 unless stated otherwise.
- Always start and end with a backstitch when sewing a seam.
- Important: please trace all relevant templates; do not cut directly from the pattern sheet.

YOU WILL NEED

- Two Fat Eighths (9 x 22in/22.75 x 56cm), for the front and lining of the mask – we've used Leafy in Green from Solstice by Sally Kelly for Windham Fabrics for the front, and Prince Paisley from Solstice by Sally Kelly for Windham Fabrics for the lining
- One 5 x 12in (12.75 x 30.5cm) piece of fusible fleece, for the padding – we've used Vlieseline H640
- One 16in (40.75cm) length of ½in (1.25cm) wide elastic, for the sleep mask strap
- Safety pin
- Blunt needle or bodkin
- Sleep Mask templates A and B on Pattern Sheet C
- All-purpose or 40wt thread in a colour that coordinates with both the front and lining fabrics

CUTTING INSTRUCTIONS

From the front fabric:

- One Sleep Mask A piece, making sure that your fabric is the right way up if it is directional (there is a top and bottom to the pattern) and the grain line arrow is parallel to the lengthwise grain (see pages 122, 123 and 140); mark all notches
- One 2 x 20in (5 x 50.75cm) strip for the elastic casing

From the lining fabric:

- One Sleep Mask A piece, making sure that your fabric is the right way up if it is directional and the grain line arrow is parallel to the lengthwise grain (see pages 122, 123 and 140); mark all notches

From the fusible fleece:

- One Sleep Mask B piece; mark both notches

Using silk

For a luxurious finish, why not make your sleep mask with silk? People feel scared to handle silk, because it can be a little slippery, but it's so worth using: it is one of the strongest natural fibres in the world, and its lightweight and breathable properties are effective at keeping you cool. Refer to the information on page 18 for guidance on cutting it out. Silk can be very expensive, but we have a cost-saving solution: look out for vintage silk scarves or handkerchiefs in thrift/charity stores or online marketplaces to use for your mask!

METHOD

1 Centre and press the fusible fleece onto the wrong side (WS) of the sleep-mask lining piece. Note that if you wish to use Vlieseline H640, like we have, it will require an iron set to medium heat – the two dots on the iron – and a damp pressing cloth to adhere it to the fabric.

2 Fold the strip for the elastic casing in half lengthways with the right sides (RS) facing. Sew the long edges together with a ⅜in (1cm) seam allowance, backstitching at the beginning and end of your seam, and making sure to leave long thread tails at the start (this will help you turn through the casing in the next step). Trim the seam allowance down to ⅛in (3mm); this will reduce bulk inside the casing, and make threading the elastic through later much easier.

3 Thread the tails of thread onto a blunt needle (or a bodkin if you have one) and tie them with a knot. Take the needle inside the elastic casing and out the other end to turn it through to the RS.

4 Roll the seam until it is centred along the length of the casing, then press the casing with an iron.

5 Cut the elastic to the required length to curve around the back of your head and fit from temple to temple while not stretched (approx. 13in/33cm). Feed it through the casing with the help of a safety pin. When the bottom end of the elastic (the end without the safety pin) matches the open raw edge of the casing you entered, pin it in place. Then carry on feeding through the rest of the elastic, all the way along, until the safety pin end matches the open raw edge at the other end of the casing. Pin this in place too.

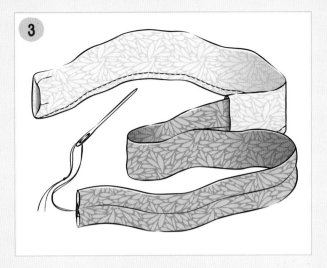

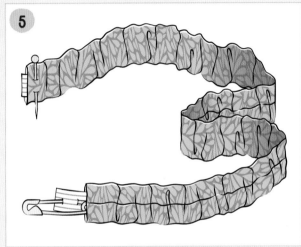

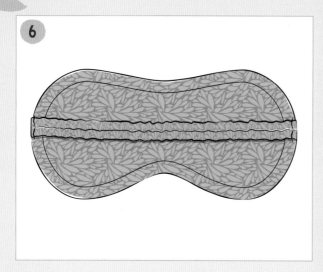

6 Using the two side notches to help with alignment, pin the strap over the sleep mask front, ensuring its seam faces upwards and is level with the side notches. Baste/tack the ends of the strap to the sides of the mask with a ¼in (5mm) seam allowance, backstitching a couple of times for security. Remove the pins.

7 Place the lining piece on top of the front, RS facing and with the strap sandwiched inside. Pin in place.

8 Starting at one of the two lower notches, sew the lining and front piece together, following the edge of the fusible fleece as a guide and working around the outside, across the top and all the way around to the other lower notch. This leaves a gap near the nose area for you to turn the mask right side out.

9 To ensure the curved seams turn through neatly, approximately every 1in (2.5cm) cut small notches into the seam allowance, being careful not to get too close to the stitches. Trim the seam allowance to ¼in (5mm) deep. Turn the mask through to the RS then press with an iron. If you've used silk for the mask, remember to set the iron to a silk setting to avoid leaving scorch marks!

10 Turn the raw edges of the gap to the inside, then close the opening by hand with ladder stitch (see page 126). Put your sleep mask on and relax!

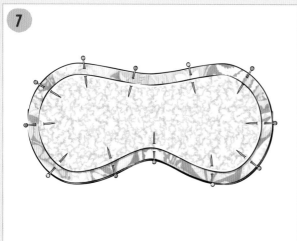

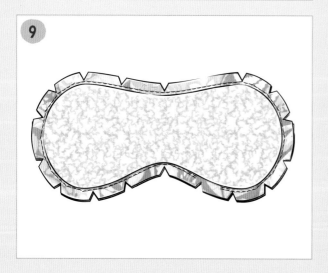

OPPOSITE:
Top mask – Front is Prince Paisley from Solstice by Sally Kelly for Windham Fabrics, strap is Leafy in Fuchsia from Solstice by Sally Kelly for Windham Fabrics.
Bottom mask – Blake Silk Satin by Liberty™.

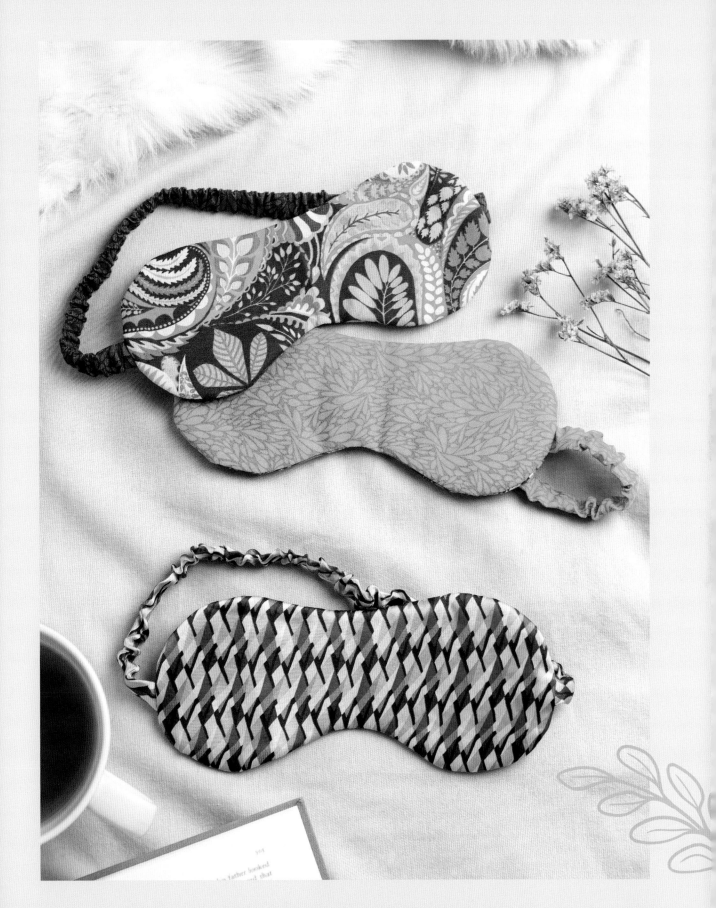

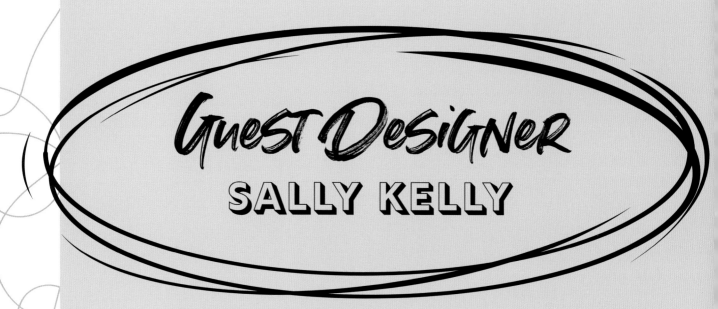

GUEST DESIGNER
SALLY KELLY

We are incredibly excited to introduce you to the wonderful world of Sally Kelly, which is always brimming with exquisite patterns and swirling colours from across the spectrum. Prepare to find yourself in fantastical landscapes with blooming flowers, wonders of the natural world, and charming creatures, all in hues that are guaranteed to lift your spirits. The level of detail is incredible, and you never get bored when sewing with them; there is always something new to discover.

Sally was a senior designer at Liberty™ for many years before setting up her own studio in London. She now produces bespoke prints for the home (and our studio walls) and gorgeous collections for Windham Fabrics.

In the past, we have used her quilting cottons for patchwork and garments, and her heavier canvas for aprons and bags. For this book's sleep mask, we chose a couple of our favourite cotton prints from her Solstice range, but have loved every one of her collections for Windham so be sure to add her to your *Menopause Makes* inspiration list.

Jenni & Kay x

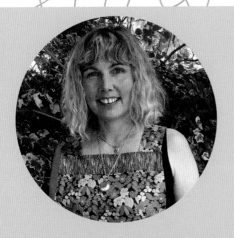

A Few Words From Sally:

'Going through menopause is an emotional time and the feeling of anxiety, at times, can be overwhelming. Spending time with your female friends experiencing similar circumstances can be a great source of comfort, and doing a mindful activity like sewing is something you can do together. Pick a simple project and then enjoy the pleasure of stitching. Sewing is a wonderful way to express and explore your creative side; every make will have a story behind it, and will always evoke very special memories of the time you spent making it.

The projects for *Menopause Makes* give you the perfect opportunity to enjoy the process of sewing, and have something precious to love at the end. I never go to bed without my sleepmask since discovering its benefits. I sleep so much better as a result, and it helps to switch off the world and take me into a deep and long rest. It's a perfect gift to make for a friend and show her you care.'

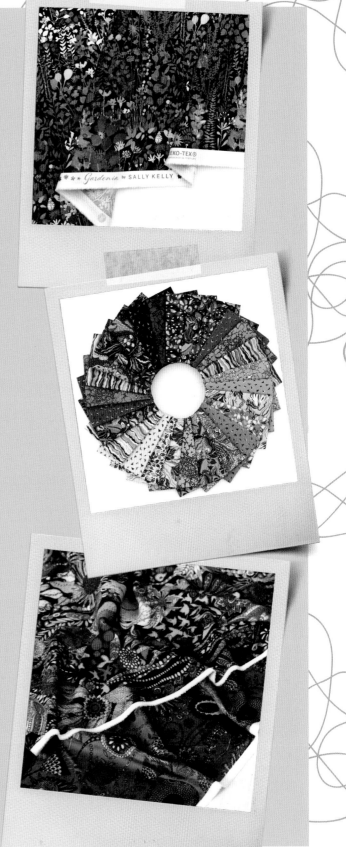

Symptom #2
MEMORY LOSS

With menopause comes a natural decline in oestrogen.
This hormone contributes to many things,
including memory performance.

So, it is hardly surprising that some of us women lose track of
what we have put where. Is your mobile phone in the fridge or in
a drawer somewhere, and who has hidden the car keys AGAIN?

We form emotional attachments to things we make with our own hands,
and so the act of sewing your very own basket will cement this little
container in your memory, and help you remember it as a safe, consistent
spot to deposit all your daily essentials.

This project allows for playful fabric choices, so have fun selecting different
fabrics for both the inside and outside of the basket.

BASKET FOR LOST THINGS

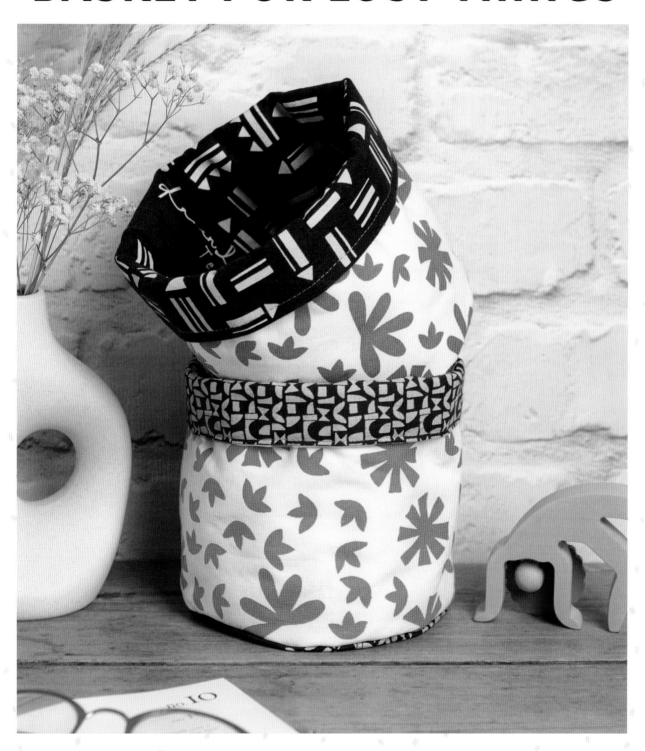

DIFFICULTY RATING

FINISHED SIZE

5in (12.75cm) diameter, 5in (12.75cm) tall

NOTES

- All seam allowances are ½in (1.25cm) unless stated otherwise.
- Sew using a stitch length of 2.4 unless stated otherwise.
- Always start and end with a backstitch when sewing a seam.
- Important: please trace all relevant templates; do not cut directly from the pattern sheet.

YOU WILL NEED

- One Fat Eighth (9 x 22in/22.75 x 56cm), for the outer fabric – OR see alternative in second bullet
- One Fat Quarter (22 x 18in/56 x 45.75cm) that coordinates with the outer fabric, for the lining fabric **OR** Two 18 x 14in (45.75 x 35.75cm) pieces of printed cotton, for the outer and lining fabrics – we've used Meadow in neon pink on white by Karen Lewis for the outer, and Improv in light blue on navy by Karen Lewis for the lining
- One 27½ x 6in (70 x 15.25cm) piece of fusible interfacing, to add structure – we've used Vlieseline H250
- One 16½ x 6in (42 x 15.25cm) piece of fusible fleece, for the padding – we've used Vlieseline H640
- All-purpose or 40wt thread to match or deliberately contrast with the lining fabric (note: this colour will be visible on the outside of the finished basket)
- Basket for Lost Things templates A and B on Pattern Sheet C

CUTTING INSTRUCTIONS

From the outer fabric:

- One 17½ x 7in (45.5 x 17.75cm) piece, for the basket sides

From the lining fabric:

- Two 6¼in (16cm) diameter circles, using template A, for the bases
- One 17½ x 7in (45.5 x 17.75cm) piece, for the basket sides

From the fusible interfacing:

- Two 5¼in (13.5cm) diameter circles, using template B, for the bases
- One 16½ x 6in (42 x 15.25cm) piece, for the lining basket side

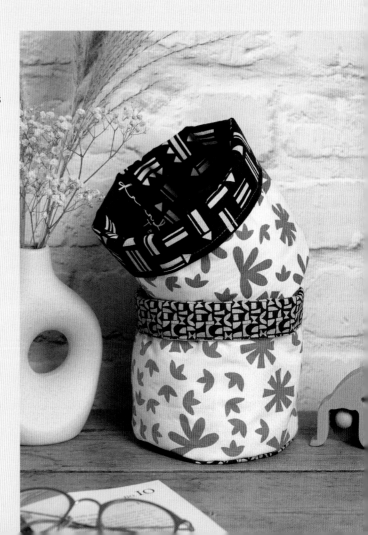

METHOD

1 Centre an interfacing circle – shiny side down – onto the wrong side (WS) of each base circle, ensuring there's a ½in (1.25cm) seam allowance all around the outside. Fuse in place with an iron. If you are using Vlieseline H250 like we have, you will need to use a dry iron on the silk/wool setting – the single dot on the iron – for around 8 seconds. Repeat with the rectangular pieces of lining fabric and interfacing.

2 Repeat Step 1 with the fusible fleece and outer rectangle piece. If you are using Vlieseline H640 like we have, you will need to set the iron to a medium heat – the two dots on the iron – and use a damp pressing cloth to help the fleece adhere to the fabric.

3 Pin or clip the shorter ends of the lining rectangle right sides (RS) together. Sew with a ½in (1.25cm) seam allowance. Remove the pins or clips, then press the seam allowance open. Repeat with the outer rectangle. These are your basket sides.

4 Fold the top edge of the outer fabric basket side to the WS by ½in (1.25cm), and press in place. Repeat with the lining fabric.

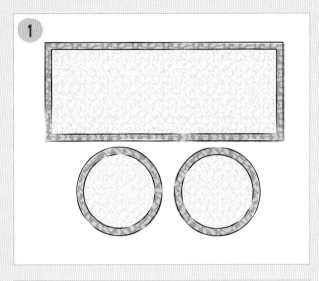

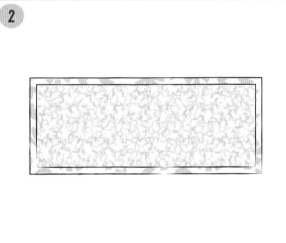

Directional fabric

If your lining fabric is directional, in Step 4 you will want to fold along the bottom edge rather than the top; this is so, when you fold over the cuff at the end, the fabric will be the right way up on the outside of the basket.

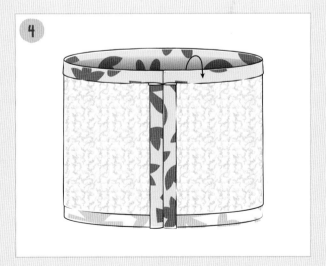

5 Use pins to mark the quarter-way points around the edges of the two circles, and along the bottom (unfolded) edges of the lining and outer fabric basket sides. Note that the seam on the two side pieces can be one quarter-way point.

6 Pin or clip one base circle to the bottom edge of the lining fabric, RS together and lining up the quarter-way points. With the circle uppermost, stitch the two pieces together with a ½in (1.25cm) seam allowance, using the edge of the interfacing as a guide. (See also the tip below.) Trim the seam allowances so that they measure ¼in (5mm).

7 Repeat Step 6 with the remaining base circle and outer side piece. Turn out so the RS of the fabric is on the outside.

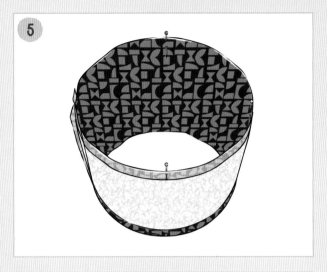

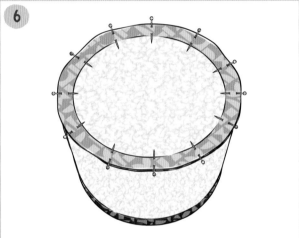

Stitching circles

When machine sewing around a curve, as you do in Steps 6 and 7, we recommend going slowly. Every 5 or 6 stitches, leave the needle down, lift the presser foot and rotate the fabric to ease around the curve.

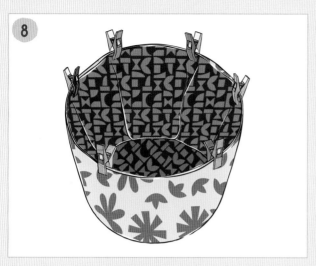

8 Place the lining inside the outer, WS together and matching the side seams. Pin or clip all around, aligning the top folded-over edges.

9 Sew the two basket pieces together using edge-stitch, with a seam allowance of approx. ⅛in (3mm) and a stitch length of 3.0. (See page 125 for more information on edge-stitching.) Start stitching just before the side seam, for a neater finish. If you use the free arm of your machine (you may need to remove the flatbed section to reveal this), you can wrap the basket around this and make sewing this step much easier.

10 Fold over a cuff of approx. 1½in (3.75cm) to reveal your lining fabric. Give a gentle press if required.

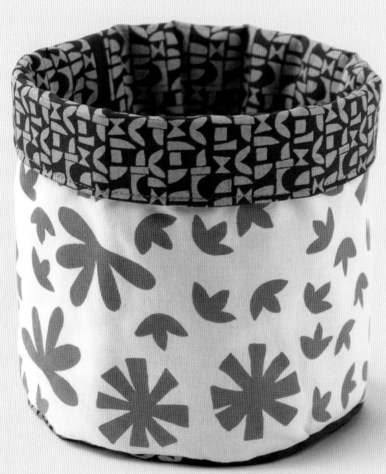

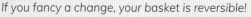

If you fancy a change, your basket is reversible!

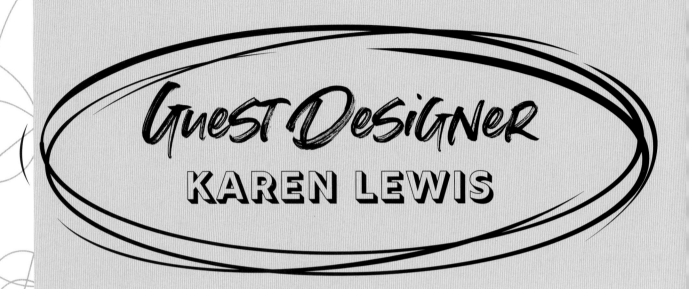

GUEST DESIGNER
KAREN LEWIS

Karen Lewis is an inspiring maker who switched up careers in her early forties to delve into printmaking and quilting. She now teaches all over the world, has written two books, and has many gorgeous fabric prints with her name on the selvedge.

We love her confident colour choices, her laid-back aesthetic and how she supports creative students with online courses and in-person retreats. We are delighted to include her hand screen-printed panels in our Basket for Lost Things and hope that you enjoy her work as much as we do!

Jenni & Kay X

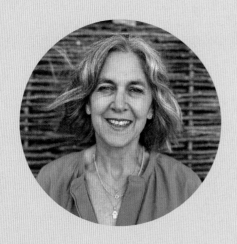

A Few Words from Karen:

'Entering and living through menopause
is a challenging time for women.
Not only might we suffer from all sorts of
symptoms but life is at a real peak, being
sandwiched between aging parents and
demanding older children. My main symptoms
have been emotional ones including increased
anxiety – organizing things I would have done
normally in the blink of an eye gets me all
anxious! Crafting has been an absolute godsend
for me at this time, enabling me to switch off
from the stresses around me, giving me calmness
and mindfulness. Sewing as a pastime has so
many valuable qualities, and it is never too late
to give it a try and feel the benefits of wellness
from engaging in it.'

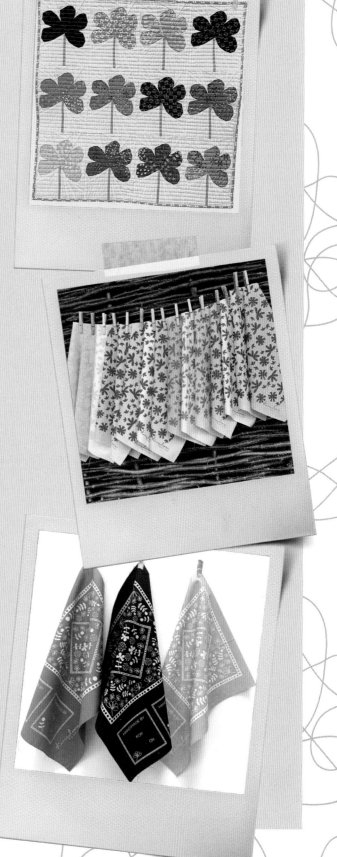

SYMPTOM #3
LOW MOOD

Hormonal changes during the menopause can affect both your physical and mental health. Feelings of sadness, low mood and depression can begin to take over your general emotional state, and it can be hard to focus on the future or plan something to look forward to.

A change of scenery can help spark positive feelings, whether you choose to be in your own company or seek that of family and friends. Our Weekend-away Tote is a stress-free project to work on in anticipation of your well-deserved time out, and to take with you when your adventure starts.

The simple construction (no zips or fasteners needed) means you can focus your energy on creative fabric and strap choices to reflect your personality and flair. There's a handy pocket inside for storing essentials like keys, phones and tissues when you need a good cry! They may well be tears of joy if you are heading off somewhere exciting, feeling super proud of your me-made creation.

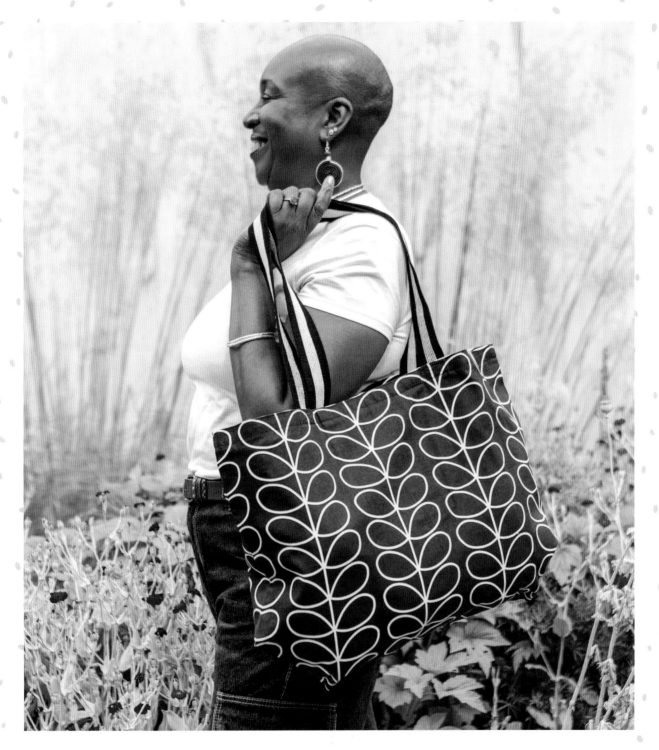

WEEKEND-AWAY TOTE

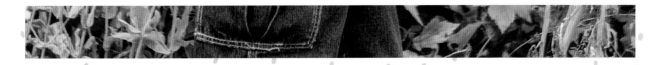

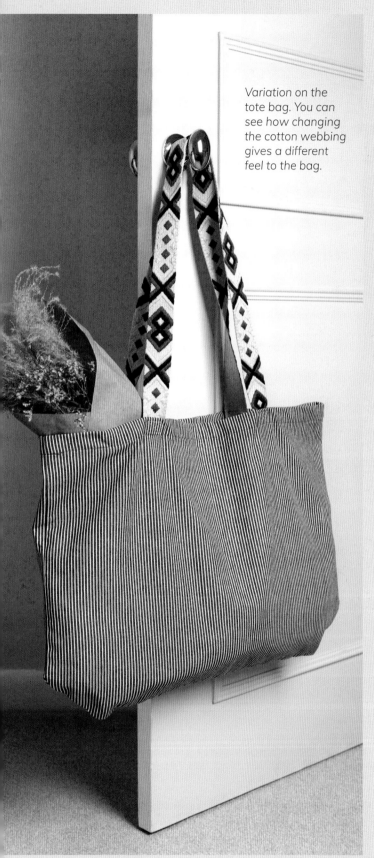

Variation on the tote bag. You can see how changing the cotton webbing gives a different feel to the bag.

DIFFICULTY RATING

FINISHED SIZE

Not including straps:
23 x 16½in (58.5 x 42cm)

Including straps:
23 x 23½in (58.5 x 59.75cm)

NOTES

- All seam allowances are ½in (1.25cm) unless stated otherwise.
- Sew using a stitch length of 2.4 unless stated otherwise.
- Always start and end with backstitch when sewing a seam.

YOU WILL NEED

- One 20in (50cm) length of 54in (140cm) wide upholstery weight fabric, for the bag sides – we used Orla Kiely Furnishing Cotton Fabric Linear Stem in Whale Blue for the main fabric
- One 8in (20.5cm) wide x 19in (48.25cm) piece of medium-weight cotton fabric, for the pocket – we used Cotton Denim Hickory Stripe in Denim Blue and White (this was also used for the bag sides of the variation, left)
- One 71in (180.5cm) length of approx. 1½in (4cm) wide cotton webbing, for the straps
- Size 90/14 universal sewing-machine needle
- All-purpose or 40wt cotton thread, to match the bag fabric

CUTTING INSTRUCTIONS

From the bag sides fabric:
- Two 24in (61cm) wide x 19in (48.25cm) tall pieces

From the webbing:
- Two 35½in (90cm) lengths

METHOD

MAKING THE POCKET

1 Along the shorter ends of the pocket rectangle, turn under double hems: turn the edge to the wrong side (WS) by ½in (1.25cm) then another ½in (1.25cm). Pin or clip, press and sew ⅜in (1cm) from the outer fold. (For more information on stitching hems, see page 128.)

2 Fold over the top (short) edge of the fabric by 3in (7.75cm), right sides (RS) facing, and press. Fold over the bottom edge by 6in (15.25cm) and press. There will be a 1in (2.5cm) overlap. Clip or pin together, particularly around the overlap.

3 Sew the sides, through all the layers, with a ½in (1.25cm) seam allowance. Reinforce the stitching at the overlap by going over it a couple of times.

4 Turn the pocket RS out, press and set aside. You can add a label to your pocket at this point if you wish (see pages 142–143).

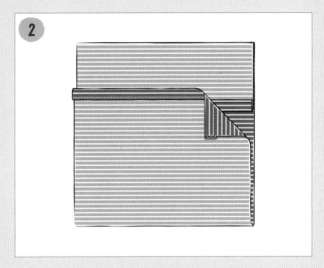

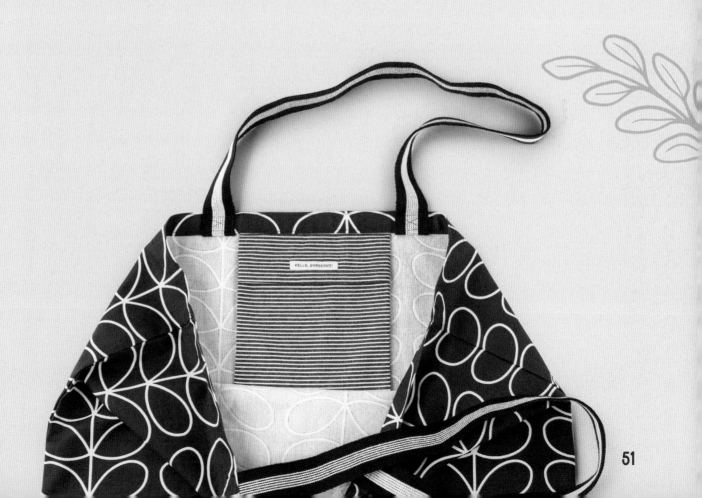

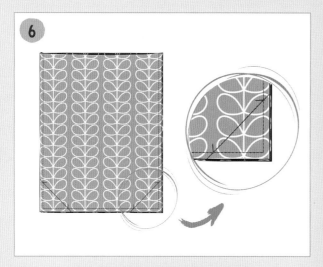

MAKING THE BAG

5 Place the two bag panels RS together. Sew along the sides and the bottom only with a ½in (1.25cm) seam allowance, pivoting at the corners (see page 127 for more information).

6 From the seams made in Step 5, mark points that are 4in (10cm) up from the bottom seam and 4in (10cm) across from the side seams. Join the two marks at each side, creating two diagonal, 45-degree lines. Sew along each line.

7 Trim away the corners, ½in (1.25cm) away from the stitch lines (see page 128).

8 To finish the seam allowances, sew the side, diagonal and bottom edges with overcast stitch (see page 125), starting at one top edge and working round to the other. Press the side seam allowances in one direction.

FINISHING

9 Turn over the top edge of the bag by ½in (1.25cm) and press. Turn over again by 1in (2.5cm) and press. Pin or clip in place. If you have a seam gauge, this would be very helpful at this step; it doesn't melt under the iron like a tape measure might!

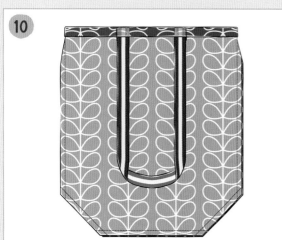

10 Allocate one side of the bag as the front (it doesn't matter which). Along the top folded edge, mark 6in (15.25cm) in from the right and left sides of the bag front. Take one strap and tuck the ends into the fold, butting the ends up to the fold, underneath your marks, the RS facing upwards, and with the 'loop' of the strap pointing downwards. Check the strap is not twisted. Pin or clip in place. Repeat with the bag back.

11 On the bag back, position the pocket centrally between the straps, tucking its top edge into the fold (see the photograph on page 51). Pin or clip in place.

12 Starting at a side seam, stitch all around the top of the bag, close to the loose edge of the fold, with a stitch length of 3.0. Make sure you don't stitch the bag closed when you do this!

13 Stitch a second line of stitching, close to the top edge of the bag (this is known as edge-stitching, see page 125) to add a smart finish.

14 Fold up the straps so they are the right way up. Use a water-soluble fabric marker to draw a rectangle on the WS of the strap, within the stitch lines of the fold and roughly the same width as the strap. Sew around the rectangle a couple of times to secure the strap in place, then sew a cross inside (see the photograph, below) for strength and extra security.

15 Turn the bag through to the RS. Poke out the corners using a point turner or another blunt-ended tool (like a chopstick, but nothing sharp like scissors!). Press the corners and all seams.

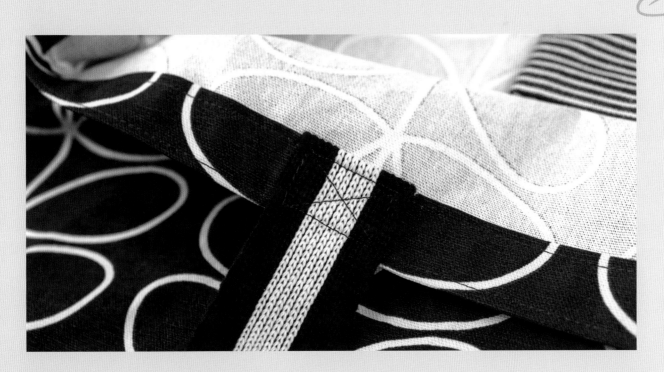

Symptom #4

DRY, ITCHY SKIN

A plummet in hormones often results in menopausal skin and hair changes (as if it wasn't bad enough first time around during adolescence!). Dry and itchy skin is one of the most common symptoms that women experience during menopause, along with other skin changes such as redness and flushing, spots and acne. Hair may thin, change its texture and become dry, whereas facial hair can thicken and appear more visible.

The great news is that these symptoms can be alleviated with specialist lotions and potions and getting into a good habit of moisturizing and conditioning is one positive change that can really help.

Why not store these new essentials in a beautiful pouch that can be moved from bathroom to bedroom and look stylish on your travels too. This project will fill you with pride as you smash the challenge of inserting a zip and stitch a functional and modern pouch – or multiple pouches for all of your products. You can even have a go with waterproof fabrics for a really professional finish.

ZIPPED POTION POUCH

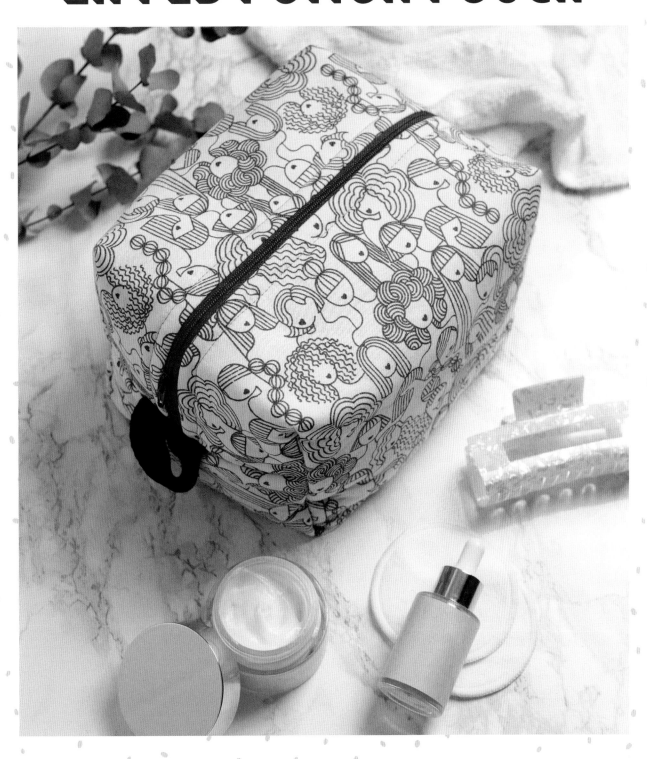

DIFFICULTY RATING

FINISHED SIZE

8in (20.25cm) wide x 6in (15.25cm) deep
x 5in (12.75) high

NOTES

- All seam allowances are ¼in (5mm) unless stated otherwise.
- Sew using a stitch length of 2.4 unless stated otherwise.
- Always start and end with backstitch when sewing a seam.
- The width-of-fabric (WOF) measurements assume you are cutting from a bolt measuring 44in (112cm) wide; check the width of the bolt when purchasing your own fabric.

YOU WILL NEED

- One ½yd x WOF (18 x 44in/45.75 x 112cm) of outer fabric – we've used Linear Sup Ladies in Playful by Rashida Coleman-Hale for Ruby Star Society
- One ½yd x WOF (18 x 44in/45.75 x 112cm) of lining fabric – we used a medium-weight cotton in blue
- One ½yd x WOF (18 x 44in/45.75 x 112cm) of fusible interfacing – we used Vlieseline H250
- One ½yd x WOF (18 x 44in/45.75 x 112cm) of fusible fleece – we used Vlieseline H640
- One 16in (41cm) zip – avoid one with metal teeth, as we'll be cutting the ends off
- One 12in (30.5cm) length of 1in (2.5cm) wide woven tape
- All-purpose or 40wt thread to the match the outer fabric
- All-purpose or 40wt thread to match the lining fabric

CUTTING INSTRUCTIONS

From the outer fabric:
- Two 14 x 12in (35.5 x 30.5cm) pieces

From the lining fabric:
- Two 14 x 12in (35.5 x 30.5cm) pieces

From the fusible interfacing:
- Two 14 x 12in (35.5 x 30.5cm) pieces

From the fusible fleece:
- Two 14 x 12in (35.5 x 30.5cm) pieces

From the woven tape:
- Two 6in (15.25cm) lengths

Stashbusting!

The fabric amounts listed for this project assume you are buying fabric specially for your pouch, but if you have a fabric stash, see what you need in the cutting instructions – you may already have enough.

METHOD

1 Press the fusible fleece onto the wrong side (WS) of each outer fabric rectangle. Note that if you wish to use Vlieseline H640, it will require an iron set to medium heat – the two dots on the iron – and a damp pressing cloth to help adhere it to the fabric.

2 Press the fusible interfacing onto the WS of the lining fabric rectangles. Note that if you wish to use Vlieseline H250, as we have, it will require a dry iron on a silk/wool setting – one dot on the iron – and you will need to press for around 8 seconds.

3 With the zip-slider side of the zip facing the right side (RS) of the fabric, centre the zip along the top edge of one of the outer pieces and clip together. Note that the length of the zip will mean it overhangs at each side of the outer piece by approx. 1in (2.5cm). Make sure the zip is closed, with the zip slider pulled completely to one end of the zip.

4 Attach the zipper foot to your machine. Baste/tack the zip in place using a long 4.0 stitch length and with an ⅛in (3mm) seam allowance.

5 Place one of the lining pieces over the stitched outer piece, RS facing and aligning all the outer edges. The zip should be sandwiched between the two fabrics. Clip the layers together. Sew together along the top edge with a ¼in (5mm) seam allowance, using a regular stitch length of around 2.4. Once sewn, flip the pieces so that they are WS together.

Note: The line on the zip tape where the texture changes is normally ¼in (5mm) from the edge of the zip, although you won't be able to see this transition when sewing in Step 5. You may find it helpful to draw your ¼in (5mm) seam allowance onto the WS of the lining fabric before sewing, so you can follow it with your needle.

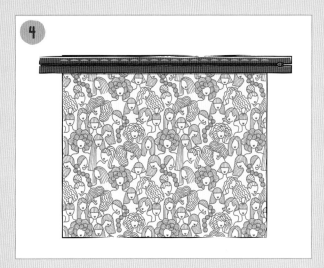

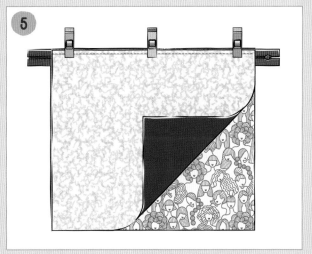

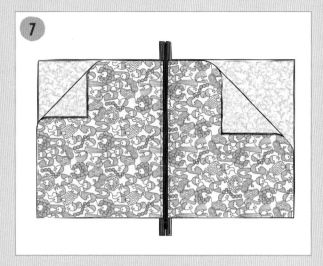

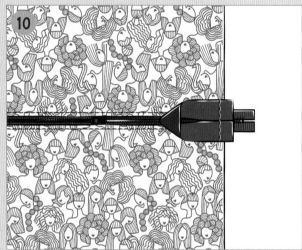

6 Repeat Steps 3–5 with the remaining outer and lining pieces, this time along the other edge of the zip. From the RS of the fabric, press the outer and lining pieces away from the zip tape.

7 With the outer fabric facing up and using matching thread, top-stitch along both sides of the zip with a 3.0 stitch length (see page 125), sewing ¼in (5mm) away from the zip teeth (use the zipper-foot edge as a guide; it should be at ¼in or 5mm).

8 With the outer fabric still facing up, fold one woven tape piece in half and centre it over the bottom end of the zip (the end with the stopper). The ends of the tape should overhang by ½in (1.25cm), its edges should butt together in the middle of the zip teeth, and the 'loop' of the tape should face inwards (refer to the illustration below left as a guide to placement). Clip in place.

9 Repeat with the second tape piece on the other end of the zip. Note that you must open the zip, and pull the zip slider to the middle, before adding the tape to this end; otherwise, you may accidentally trim off the zip slider later!

10 Attach the regular foot to your machine. Using a 2.4 stitch length and ¼in (5mm) seam allowance, sew the tape pieces in place. When sewing across the end of the zip that's open, use your left hand to hold the zip teeth together as you stitch. Trim away the excess zip tape on either side of the pouch so it's flush with the sides of the fabric. Leave the zip open.

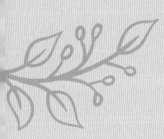

11 Match outer piece to outer piece and lining piece to lining piece, RS together, then clip or pin. Stitch the outers together along the bottom edge (see the left-hand side of the illustration) with a ½in (1.25cm) seam allowance. Repeat with the lining pieces (see the right-hand side of the illustration), but leave a 6in (15.25cm) gap in the centre of the seam (you could mark this gap if you wish). Press the seam allowances open.

12 Arrange the layers of fabric, so that the newly stitched seam of the outer is centred above the zip, and the lining seam below it. Press then clip in place at both open edges. Make sure the tabs are hidden inside (these are shown in the illustration with a transparent effect for context), on top of the zip. Sew along both open edges with a ½in (1.25cm) seam allowance, going backwards and forwards over the zip section a couple of times to add strength. At the corners, trim away a little of the seam at an angle (see page 128), being careful not to cut too close to the stitching.

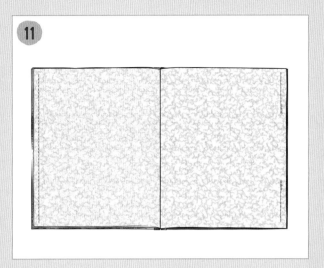

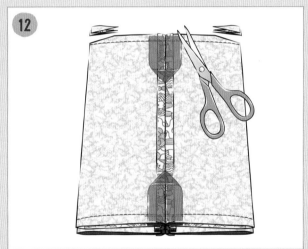

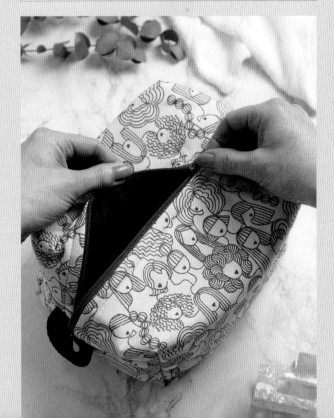

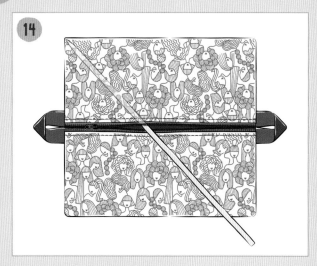

13 Through the gap, turn the lining to the RS. Ease open the zip and then turn through the zip so the pouch is RS out.

14 Poke out the corners using a point turner or another blunt-ended tool (like a chopstick, but nothing sharp like scissors!). Give the pouch a gentle press.

15 Turn the pouch inside out, so the lining is on the outside. Poke out the corners and give it a press once again.

16 Switch to a thread that matches the lining fabric. With a seam allowance of about ⅛in (3mm), sew the opening in the lining closed.

17 Now to make the pouch '3D': flatten out one of the corners to create a triangle, with the seam sitting in the centre on top of the triangle. Draw a line 2½in (6.25cm) away from the corner, then sew along the drawn line. Repeat for the three remaining corners.

18 Turn the pouch through the zip so it's RS out. Poke out the corners; the triangles will sit to the sides on the inside of the pouch and help to create extra stability.

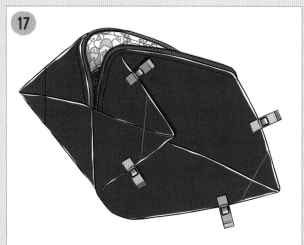

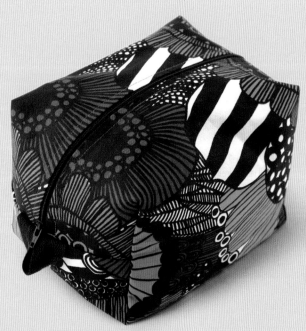

Use waterproof fabrics for your pouch for easy cleaning! If the oilcloth is structured, you could skip using fusible fleece and interfacing entirely. We used Siirtolapuutarha oilcloth by Marimekko.

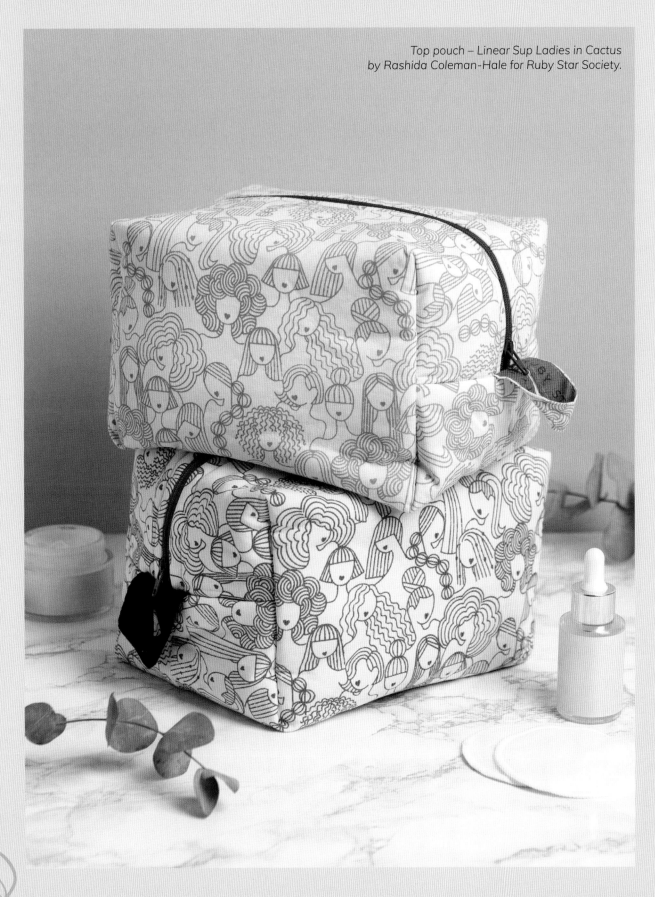

Guest Designer
RASHIDA COLEMAN-HALE

Rashida's designs have always brought a smile to our faces. Her incredible skill in combining graphic simplicity with a sense of nostalgia, and her extraordinary colour palettes, results in prints that feel cool and contemporary. We have made patchworks and garments with her fabrics through the years, and are delighted to feature them in the Log Cabin Placemats and our Zipped Potion Pouch. We are over the moon that Rashida has also designed the cover of this very book, and injected it with the fun and colour she's known for.

Rashida is one of five designers who make up the Ruby Star Society, a female-led fabric design company. They describe themselves as 'a sisterhood of empowered women who have stood together, grown strong, and learned – trial by fire – that if you tune out all the noise, listen to your inner voice and get out of your own way, you can create fearlessly.' We encourage you all to take the time to discover their designs and can't wait to see how you use them creatively in your menopause projects.

Jenni & Kay x

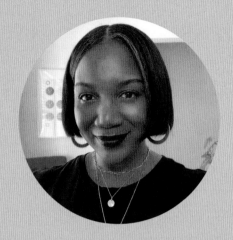

A Few Words from Rashida:

'At 48 years old, I'm not quite there yet, but I know menopause is on the horizon. I like to view it as another phase where we can continue to grow and thrive. During times like these, creativity – whether it's sewing, crafting, or designing – becomes even more important.

When menopause brings changes that can shake our confidence, creating something with our hands can ground us and bring joy. It's a way to remind ourselves that, even as our bodies go through a shift, our ability to create, express ourselves, and find happiness doesn't change. By embracing our creativity, we can stay confident and empowered as we navigate this new stage of life.'

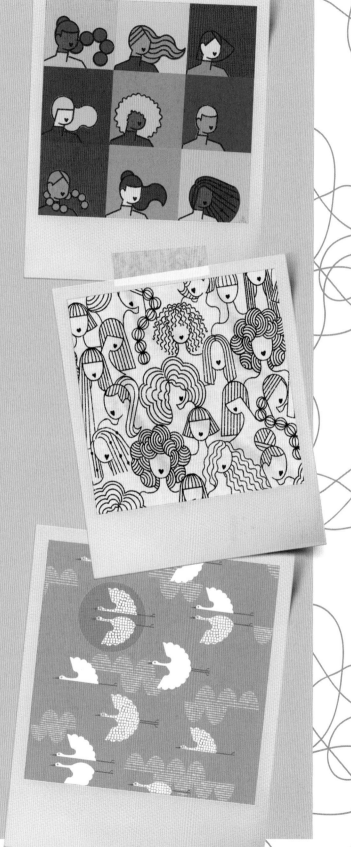

Symptom #5

STESS

Mid-life brings many challenges but throw menopausal symptoms into the mix and stress levels can rise significantly. This can manifest into a busy mind that can't switch off, and may also lead to overwhelm or loss of self-control. So how to find calm?

Numerous studies show that sewing is a mindful activity. As you focus on each stitch, you become absorbed in the moment and slow down. Once immersed in this flow of creativity, you are more likely to process stressful thoughts in an effective way.

These placemats can be constructed by hand with a needle and thread, making them very portable and therefore allowing you to find a creative respite wherever you may need it (during a break at work, in the waiting room, on the train, and so on). Even 10 to 15 minutes of stitching will make your project grow and still your mind. These placemats, which feature the traditional Log Cabin design, can be used to adorn your table and bring some handmade joy into your daily life.

Once you realize how relaxing hand sewing can be, why not try a different colour palette for every season?

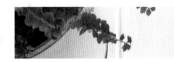

LOG CABIN PLACEMATS

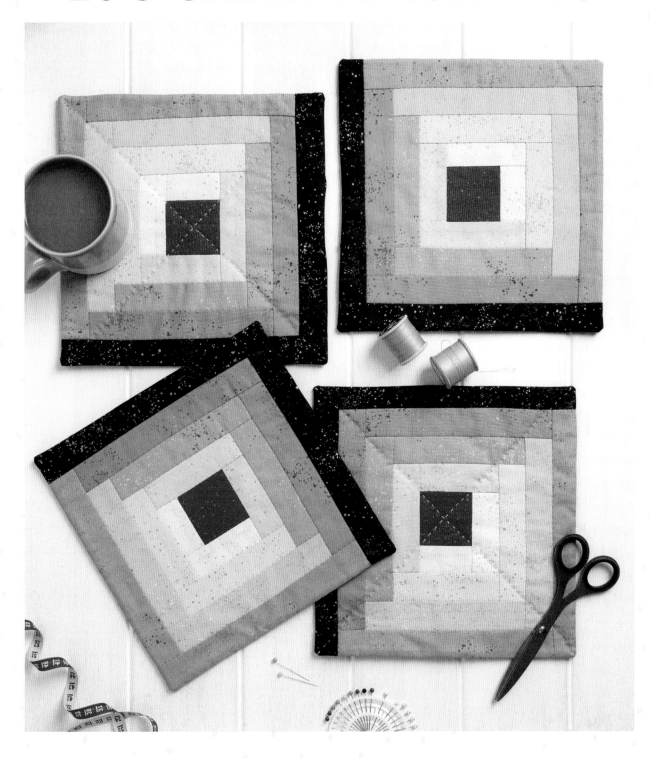

DIFFICULTY RATING

FINISHED SIZE

Each mat is 10in (25.5cm) square

NOTES

- All seam allowances are ¼in (5mm) unless stated otherwise.
- The width-of-fabric (WOF) measurements assume you are cutting from a bolt measuring 44in (112cm) wide; check the width of the bolt when purchasing your own fabric.
- As you are sewing by hand, it may help to draw in your seam lines before stitching with a marking tool; these should be ¼in (5mm) away from the fabric edge.
- Sew using running stitch, and aim for approximately 4–5 stitches per 1in (2.5cm).
- Knot your thread to start each line, and end with a couple of small backstitches to secure.
- If you are stitching on-the-go it is fine to finger-press rather than using an iron!
- Refer to pages 130 and 131 for information on cutting your patchwork pieces.

YOU WILL NEED

The following quantities make four mats.

Fabrics (we've used the Speckled collection by Rashida Coleman-Hale for Ruby Star; the specific colours are detailed in brackets):

- Fabric A (Scarlet/red) – one 5in (13cm) square
- Fabric B (White Gold/cream) – one 6in (15.25cm) square
- Fabric C (Polar/pale blue) – one Fat Sixteenth (9 x 11in/22.75 x 28cm)
- Fabric D (Sunlight/pale yellow) – one Fat Sixteenth (9 x 11in/22.75 x 28cm)
- Fabric E (Soft Blue/mid-blue) – one Fat Eighth (9 x 22in/22.75 x 56cm)
- Fabric F (Sunshine/yellow) – one Fat Eighth (9 x 22in/22.75 x 56cm)
- Fabric G (Bright Blue/bright blue) – one Fat Eighth (9 x 22in/22.75 x 56cm)
- Fabric H (Cactus/dark yellow) – one Fat Eighth (9 x 22in/22.75 x 56cm)
- Fabric I (Navy/navy) – one Fat Eighth (9 x 22in/22.75 x 53.25cm)

Everything else:

- 50wt cotton thread for piecing
- 12wt cotton or perle thread for hand quilting (optional)
- One ½yd x WOF (18 x 44in/45.75 x 112cm) or four 10½in (26.75cm) squares of backing fabric – please note, as this is the backing, it doesn't matter if they are all different
- One 36 x 45in (91.5 x 114cm) piece of heat-resistant batting/ wadding – we used a pack of Insul-Bright Heat Batting
- Hera marker, for creasing lines

Behind the block name

The design we've used for our placemats is the 'Log Cabin', a classic quilt block.

It's suggested that the name was inspired by the homes of the early pioneer settlers in America, which were log cabins. Traditionally, Log Cabin blocks have a red centre, which represents the hearth of the home.

CUTTING INSTRUCTIONS

From Fabric A:
- Four 2½in (6.5cm) squares

From Fabric B:
- Four 2½ x 1½in (6.5 x 3.75cm) strips
- Four 3½ x 1½in (9 x 3.75cm) strips

From Fabric C:
- Four 3½ x 1½in (9 x 3.75cm) strips
- Four 4½ x 1½in (11.5 x 3.75cm) strips

From Fabric D:
- Four 4½ x 1½in (11.5 x 3.75cm) strips
- Four 5½ x 1½in (14 x 3.75cm) strips

From Fabric E:
- Four 5½ x 1½in (14 x 3.75cm) strips
- Four 6½ x 1½in (16.5 x 3.75cm) strips

From Fabric F:
- Four 6½ x 1½in (16.5 x 3.75cm) strips
- Four 7½ x 1½in (19 x 3.75cm) strips

From Fabric G:
- Four 7½ x 1½in (19 x 3.75cm) strips
- Four 8½ x 1½in (21.5 x 3.75cm) strips

From Fabric H:
- Four 8½ x 1½in (21.5 x 3.75cm) strips
- Four 9½ x 1½in (24.25 x 3.75cm) strips

From Fabric I:
- Four 9½ x 1½in (24.25 x 3.75cm) strips
- Four 10½ x 1½in (26.75 x 3.75cm) strips

From the backing fabric:
- Four 10½in (26.75cm) squares

From the batting/wadding:
- Four 10½in (26.75cm) squares

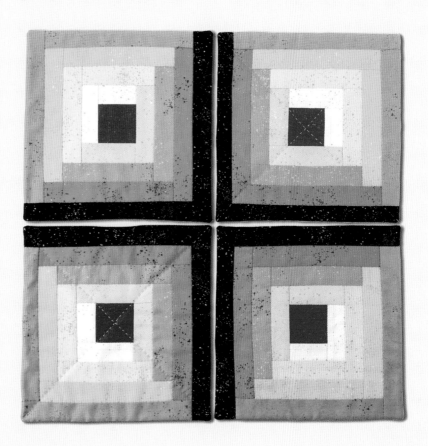

METHOD

1 To begin, place a 2½in (6.5cm) Fabric A square and 2½ x 1½in (6.5 x 3.75cm) Fabric B strip right sides (RS) together. Pin and sew together. Press the seam allowance towards the B strip.

2 With RS facing, sew a 3½ x 1½in (9 x 3.75cm) Fabric B strip to the unit made in Step 1. Press the seam allowance towards the most recently added strip.

3 With RS facing, sew a 3½ x 1½in (9 x 3.75cm) Fabric C strip to the unit made in Step 2. Press the seam allowance towards the most recently added strip.

4 With RS facing, sew a 4½ x 1½in (11.5 x 3.75cm) Fabric C strip to the unit made in Step 3. Press the seam allowance towards the most recently added strip.

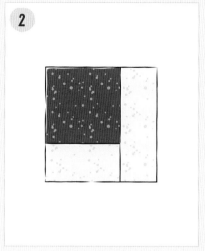

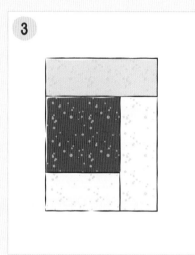

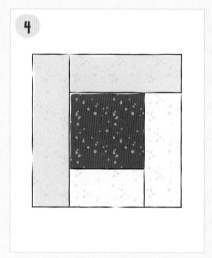

5 Following the illustration below, continue to add the strips in the following order in a counter-clockwise direction. Always press the seam allowance towards the most recently added strip.

- Fabric D – 4½ x 1½in (11.5 x 3.75cm) strip
- Fabric D – 5½ x 1½in (14 x 3.75cm) strip
- Fabric E – 5½ x 1½in (14 x 3.75cm) strip
- Fabric E – 6½ x 1½in (16.5 x 3.75cm) strip
- Fabric F – 6½ x 1½in (16.5 x 3.75cm) strip
- Fabric F – 7½ x 1½in (19 x 3.75cm) strip
- Fabric G – 7½ x 1½in (19 x 3.75cm) strip
- Fabric G – 8½ x 1½in (21.5 x 3.75cm) strip
- Fabric H – 8½ x 1½in (21.5 x 3.75cm) strip
- Fabric H – 9½ x 1½in (24.25 x 3.75cm) strip
- Fabric I – 9½ x 1½in (24.25 x 3.75cm) strip
- Fabric I – 10½ x 1½in (26.75 x 3.75cm) strip.

6 Lay out the batting/wadding square. Over this, place the backing square, RS up. Finally, centre the Log Cabin block over both layers, RS facing down. Pin or clip the three layers together.

7 Sew around all four sides, leaving a 2in (5cm) gap halfway along one of the seams for turning through.

8 Snip across the seam allowances at the corners, being careful not to cut into the seam (see page 128). Turn the placemat RS out through the gap. Poke out the corners using a point turner or another blunt-ended tool (like a chopstick, but nothing sharp like scissors!). Press the mat.

9 Close up the gap by hand with ladder stitch. (See page 126 for information on working ladder stitch.)

10 Repeat all steps to make four placemats in total.

11 This is optional: embellish your placemats by hand-quilting a cross (or any pattern you desire) across the Log-Cabin top with a heavy-weight thread such as perle cotton or 12wt cotton. You can find out more on how to do this on page 134.

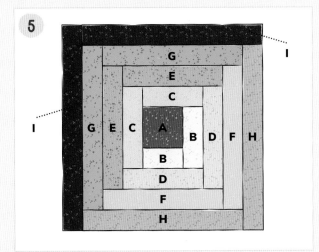

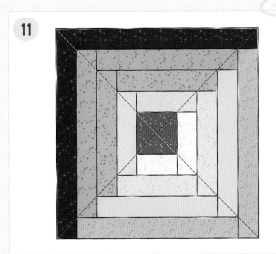

Symptom #6

BRAIN FOG

A decline in oestrogen levels can affect brain function, and a very common symptom of the menopause is brain fog. Not remembering a person's name, or the word for an everyday object, can feel especially debilitating in social situations, and can lead to low self-esteem and frustration.

Why not tackle this symptom by exercising your brain with some basic patchwork skills. The simple repetition (and a little bit of maths) involved in making quilt blocks is a good way not only to focus the brain, but to find a little calm and joy too.

Our menopausal years often coincide with major life events such as children 'flying the nest'. The classic patchwork motifs in this project are called 'Flying Geese', so it could be the perfect handmade gift for a family member or friend going off to spread their wings and embark upon a new adventure.

If you are at the beginning of your journey into patchwork and quilting, this pillow will give you the skills and confidence to later move on to sewing our beautiful Keep Cool Quilt (see page 106).

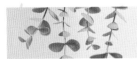

FLYING GEESE PILLOW

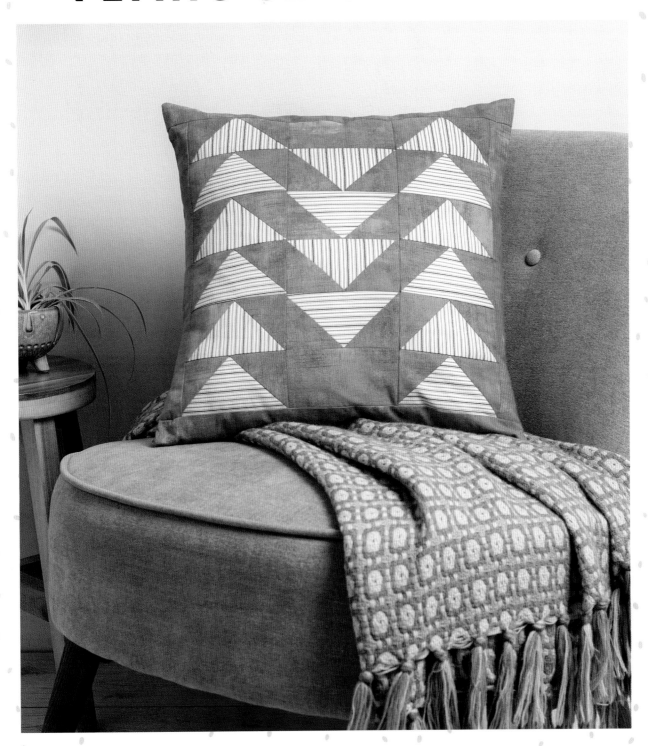

DIFFICULTY RATING

FINISHED SIZE

Finished pillow: 18in (45.75cm) square

Unfinished size of each Flying Geese block:
3 x 5½in (7.5 x 14cm)

NOTES

- All seam allowances are ¼in (5mm) unless stated otherwise.
- Sew all patchwork using a stitch length of 2.2.
- Always press from the back first then turn over and press again from the front.
- The width-of-fabric (WOF) measurements assume you are cutting from a bolt measuring 44in (112cm) wide; check the width of the bolt when purchasing your own fabric.
- Refer to pages 130 and 131 for information on cutting your patchwork pieces.

YOU WILL NEED

- One ¾yd x WOF (27 x 44in/70 x 112cm) of Fabric A, for the background – we've used Grunge in Delft Blue by Moda Fabrics
- One Fat Quarter (22 x 18in/56 x 45.75cm) of Fabric B, for the 'Geese' – this is the perfect project to upcycle a stripy shirt, which is what we have done. This makes it not only economical but also personal. Cut your fabric pieces from the shirt back and its front panels (avoiding the button plackets and pockets), and cut open the sleeves to use if necessary. Note that it's easier to cut and sew a 100% cotton shirt
- 18in (45.75cm) square pillow pad
- Marking tool, for drawing lines
- All-purpose/40wt thread, or 50wt thread

CUTTING INSTRUCTIONS

From Fabric A:

- Sixteen 3⅝in (9.25cm) squares, for bordering the 'Geese'
- Two 3 x 5½in (7.5 x 14cm) strips, as fillers
- Two 2¼ x 15½in (5.75 x 39.5cm) strips, for the side borders
- Two 2¼ x 19in (5.75 x 48.25cm) strips, for the top and bottom borders
- Two 13½ x 19in (34.25 x 48.25cm) rectangles, for the backing

From Fabric B:

- Four 6½in (16.5cm) squares

Fabric choices

We would recommend a solid fabric or non-directional print for Fabric A as this gets rotated in the finished blocks during the piecing. Stripy fabric works well for Fabric B as it gives some movement.

METHOD

MAKING THE FLYING GEESE

1 We will be using a four-at-a-time method to make our Geese. Draw a diagonal line on the wrong side (WS) of all 3⅝in (9.25cm) Fabric A squares. Place two of the squares in the top-left and bottom-right corners of a 6½in (16.5cm) Fabric B square, right sides (RS) facing and making sure that the drawn lines point in the same direction, creating one continuous diagonal line. Pin and then sew ¼in (5mm) away from each side of the drawn line.

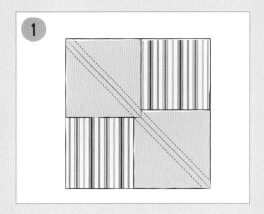

2 Cut along the drawn line to create two units. Press the seam allowances towards the smaller triangles.

3 Place another 3⅝in (9.25cm) Fabric A square over one of the Step 2 units, RS together and matching the right-angled corners. Make sure that the drawn line is in the correct orientation, pointing from the right-angled corner towards the smaller triangles. Pin and sew ¼in (5mm) away from each side of the drawn line. Cut along the drawn line.

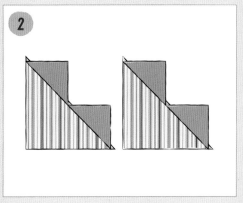

4 Press the small triangles away from Fabric B. You now have two Flying Geese blocks.

5 Repeat Steps 3 and 4 with the remaining Step 2 unit to make four Flying Geese blocks in total.

6 Repeat Steps 1–5 three more times to make 16 Flying Geese blocks in total.

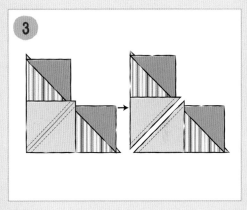

7 Trim each Flying Geese block so that it measures 3 x 5½in (7.5 x 14cm). Trim the top seam allowance first, ensuring that the distance between the point of the triangle and the top edge is ¼in (5mm). Next, trim from the bottom edge to make the unit 3in (7.5cm) deep. Then trim from the left- and right-hand sides, making sure that the large triangle sits centrally within the block (i.e. at 2¾in/7cm) and the finished block measures 5½in (14cm) wide.

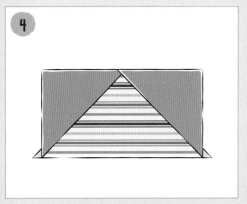

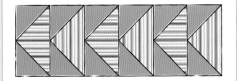

ASSEMBLING THE PILLOW

8 Sew six Flying Geese blocks into a strip. If you are using a stripy fabric like we have, alternate the direction of the stripes for each unit. Press all seam allowances in one direction, towards the base of the triangles. Repeat with six more Flying Geese blocks.

9 Repeat Step 8 with four Flying Geese blocks and two 3 x 5½in (7.5 x 14cm) strips, positioning the 3 x 5½in (7.5 x 14cm) strips at the ends, as shown in the illustration. Press the seam allowances in one direction, towards the base of the triangles.

10 Sew the three strips from Steps 8 and 9 RS together: nest the seams (see the tip below) and pin at each seam line, referring to the illustration for guidance on direction. Press the seam allowances outwards from the centre strip. This is the pillow front.

11 Rotate the pillow front, so the 'Geese' in the middle row point downwards. Pin then sew the two 2¼ x 15½in (5.75 x 39.5cm) border strips to the left- and right-hand sides of the pillow front, RS together. Press the seam allowances towards the border. Pin then sew the two 2¼ x 19in (5.75 x 48.25cm) border strips to the top and bottom of the pillow front. Press the seam allowances towards the border.

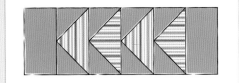

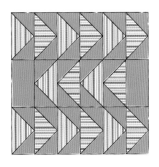

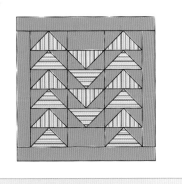

Nesting seams

This simply means pressing the seam allowance in the next row in the opposite direction to your first, so they will fit or 'nest' together and create a neat join. This allows the fabric to be evenly distributed on both sides of the seam.

12 Make a double hem along one 19in (48.25cm) side of each backing fabric rectangle: fold over the edge by ½in (1.25cm), WS facing. Press. Fold the edge again by another ½in (1.25cm) and press. Edge-stitch ⅛in (3mm) away from the folded edge (see page 125) and then press.

OPTIONAL If you wish to add a label, now is the time. We've stitched an end-fold label onto the RS of one of our backing fabric rectangles, 1½in (3.75cm) away from one long edge.

13 Lay out your finished pillow in front of you with its RS facing up. With RS together, lay a backing fabric rectangle over the pillow front, matching the raw edges at the top and sides, and with the double hem in the middle. (**Note:** if you added a label to one of the backing fabric rectangles as we have, you should use that one for this step.)

14 Lay the remaining backing fabric rectangle on the opposite side of the pillow front in the same way. The backing fabric rectangles will overlap. Pin or clip the layers together.

15 Sew around all four sides with a ½in (1.25cm) seam allowance. Trim the seam allowances at the corners at an angle to remove some of the bulk, being careful not to cut into the seam (see page 128).

16 Turn the pillow cover RS out. Poke out the corners using a point turner or another blunt-ended tool (like a chopstick, but nothing sharp like scissors!). Press, then stuff the pillow pad inside.

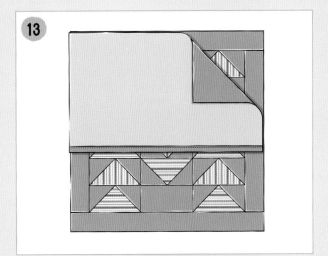

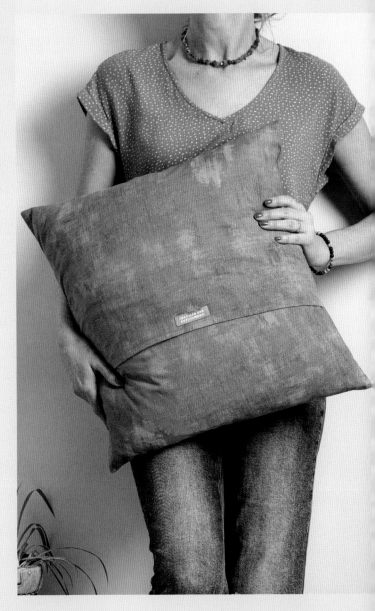

Symptom #7

ANXIETY

Feeling anxious out of the blue is perhaps one of the most surprising emotions for many menopausal women, and can frequently be misdiagnosed as depression. It is hard to articulate why you no longer feel like your usual self, but low progesterone means that you have less of your 'feel-good' hormones, and that can obviously impact your general mood. If your state of mind is altered, you can also lose perspective and become anxious over events, which may not have affected you before.

Physical symptoms of anxiety include increased heart rate and difficulty breathing. Our relaxation blanket is a tool to combat this: with its soft cotton fleece backing, it is cozy to lay beneath during yoga nidra practice, meditation or in your own quiet space.

The blanket has a patchwork front that is really fun, quick and simple to piece together, as we've used our Half Square Triangle short-cut, and then hand-tied it to the backing.

Why not select a colour palette which evokes a place in which you feel calm and happy? We have gone for a summer-garden vibe, but your blanket could be reminiscent of a beach, mountains or other favourite location.

RELAXATION BLANKET

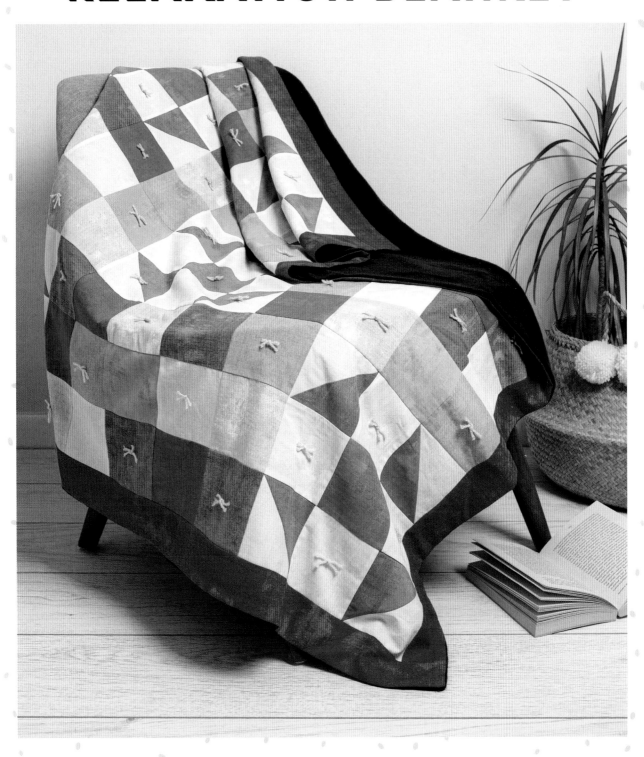

DIFFICULTY RATING

FINISHED SIZE

Finished quilt: 48½ x 64½in (123.25 x 163.75cm)

Unfinished Shoo Fly block size:
12½in (31.75cm)

Unfinished checkerboard panels:
Three-by-four panels = 12½ x 16½in (31.75 x 42cm)
Three-by-five panels = 12½ x 20½in (31.75 x 52cm)

NOTES

- All seam allowances are ¼in (5mm) unless stated otherwise.
- Sew all patchwork using a stitch length of 2.2.
- Always press from the back first then turn over and press again from the front.
- The width-of-fabric (WOF) measurements assume you are cutting from a bolt measuring 44in (112cm) wide; check the width of the bolt when purchasing your own fabric.
- Refer to pages 130 and 131 for information on cutting your patchwork pieces.

YOU WILL NEED

Fabrics (we've used the Grunge collection by Moda fabrics; specific colours are detailed in brackets):

- Fabric A (Fern/green), for the patchwork top – one ½yd x WOF (18 x 44in/45.75 x 112cm)
- Fabric B (Whisper/cream), for the patchwork top – 1yd x WOF (36 x 44in/91.5 x 112cm)
- Fabric C (Berry/dark pink), for the patchwork top – one Fat Quarter (22 x 18in or 56 x 45.75cm)
- Fabric D (Blush/pale pink), for the patchwork top – one Fat Quarter (22 x 18in/56 x 45.75cm)
- Fabric E (Sunflower/yellow), for the patchwork top – one Fat Quarter (22 x 18in/56 x 45.75cm)
- Fabric F (Sea/dark blue), for the patchwork top – one Fat Quarter (22 x 18in/56 x 45.75cm)
- Fabric G (Crystal Sea/light blue), for the patchwork top – one Fat Quarter (22 x 18in/56 x 45.75cm)
- Fabric H (Raspberry/hot pink), for the border – one ½yd x WOF (18 x 42in/45.75 x 106.75cm)

Everything else:

- One 66 x 60in (167.75 x 152.5cm) piece of wide cotton fleece, for the backing
- 50wt cotton thread for piecing and sewing
- Thick complementary- or contrasting-coloured thread for hand-tying, such as 8wt or 12wt cotton or perle thread, embroidery floss or yarn – we've used a duck-egg blue yarn
- Needle with a large enough eye for your chosen thread or yarn
- Square quilting ruler, minimum 4½in x 4½in (11.5 x 11.5cm)
- Curved safety pins
- Erasable marking tool

'Made with Love + Swear Words'

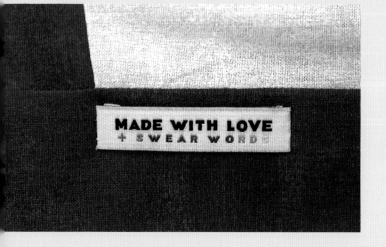

CUTTING INSTRUCTIONS

From Fabric A:

- Four 10¼in (26cm) squares
- Eight 4½in (11.5cm) squares

From Fabric B:

- Four 10¼in (26cm) squares
- Forty-five 4½in (11.5cm) squares

From Fabric C:

- Sixteen 4½in (11.5cm) squares

From Fabric D:

- Sixteen 4½in (11.5cm) squares

From Fabric E:

- Sixteen 4½in (11.5cm) squares

From Fabric F:

- Sixteen 4½in (11.5cm) squares

From Fabric G:

- Sixteen 4½in (11.5cm) squares

From Fabric H:

- Six 3in (7.5cm) wide strips x WOF

From the fleece backing:

- One 49½ x 65½ (125.75 x 166.5cm) piece

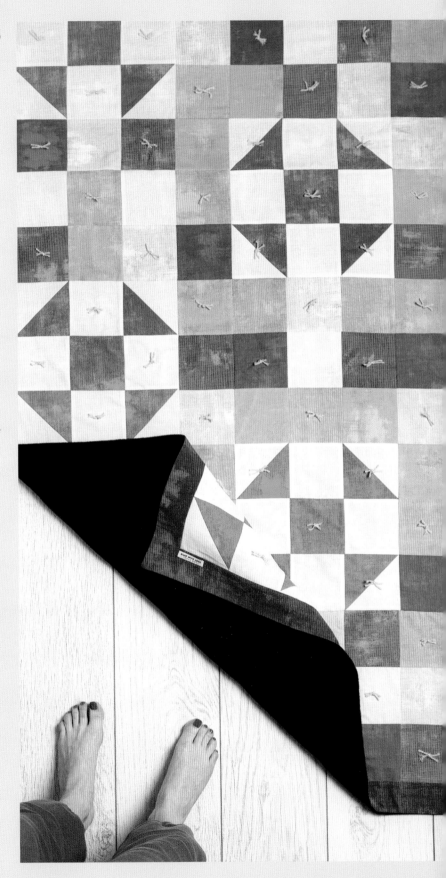

METHOD

MAKING THE HALF SQUARE TRIANGLES

1 We will be using the eight-at-a-time method to make our Half Square Triangles (HSTs). Draw two diagonal lines on the wrong side (WS) of one 10¼in (26cm) Fabric B square. Place this Fabric B square over one 10¼in (26cm) Fabric A square, right sides (RS) together, and pin. Sew ¼in (5mm) away from each side of the diagonal lines.

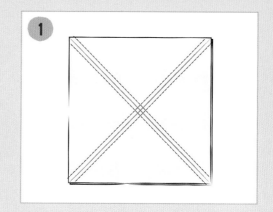

2 Cut along the drawn lines, then cut again along the horizontal and vertical halfway points to create eight HST. Press the seam allowances towards Fabric A.

3 Repeat three times to make thirty-two HSTs in total.

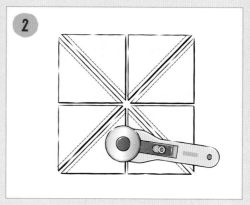

4 With a rotary cutter and ruler, trim each HST to 4½in (11.5cm) square: line up the seam with the 45-degree line on the ruler, then extend the HST slightly beyond the 4½in (11.5cm) marks on the ruler and trim any excess fabric you see extending beyond the ruler at the top and right-hand side, as shown. Rotate the block by 180 degrees, and this time line up the ruler along the bottom and left-hand edges on the 4½in (11.5cm) lines. Trim away any excess you see on the top and right-hand edges once more.

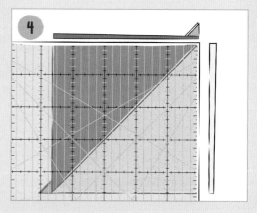

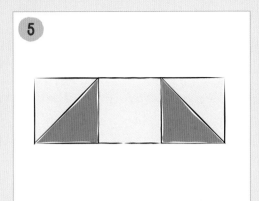

PIECING THE SHOO FLY BLOCKS

5 Sew a HST to the left-hand side of a 4½in (11.5cm) Fabric B square, RS together and with the Fabric B 'triangle' of the HST in the top-left corner. Press the seam allowance towards the Fabric B square. Sew a second HST to the right-hand side of the unit, RS together and with the Fabric B 'triangle' of the HST in the top-right corner. Press the seam allowance towards the Fabric B square, as before.

6 Repeat Step 5 to make sixteen units in total.

7 Sew two 4½in (11.5cm) Fabric B squares to the two sides of one 4½in (11.5cm) Fabric A square. Press the seam allowances towards the Fabric B squares.

8 Repeat Step 7 to make eight units in total.

9 Rotate eight of the Step 5 units so that the Fabric A 'triangles' point upwards and towards the centre square. Nesting the seams, sew each of these units to the bottom of a Step 7 unit. Sew a Step 5 unit that you haven't rotated to the top of each newly joined unit, again nesting the seams. You should have eight Shoo Fly blocks in total. Press the seam allowances towards the centre units.

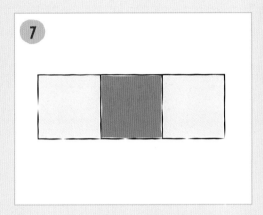

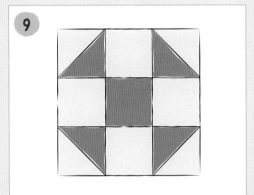

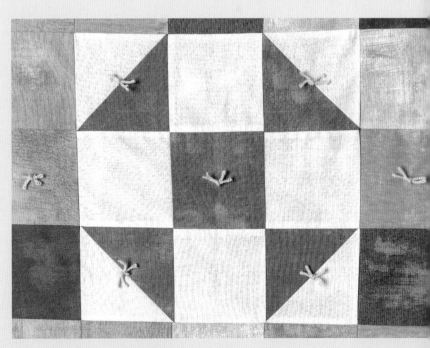

PIECING THE PATCHWORK TOP

10 Create seven checkerboard panels with the 4½in (11.5cm) coloured squares, referring to the illustration for colour placement. There are three panels made with 15 squares, and four panels made with 12 squares – the illustration below shows how the panels will be placed when the quilt top is assembled. To make each panel, sew the squares RS together in rows first. Alternate the direction in which you press the seam allowances in each row of each panel: press the seam allowances in the top row to the right, the seam allowances in the second row to the left, the seam allowances in the third row to the right, and so on. Then sew the rows RS together, nesting the seams. (We recommend pinning at each seam before sewing.)

11 Referring to the illustration, sew the Shoo Fly blocks to the units from Step 10, RS together and retaining the five separate rows as shown. Press the seam allowances away from the Shoo Fly blocks.

12 Sew the five rows RS together. Press the seam allowances downwards. Please note that not every seam will nest at this stage, but when possible try to nest them.

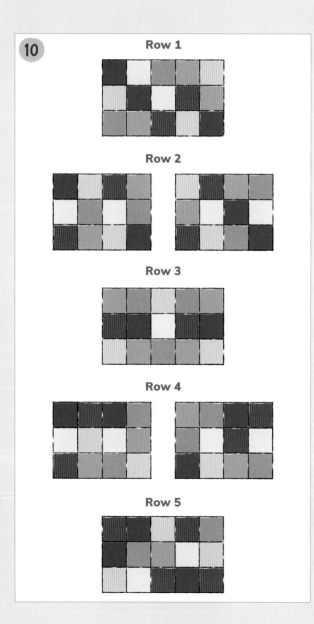

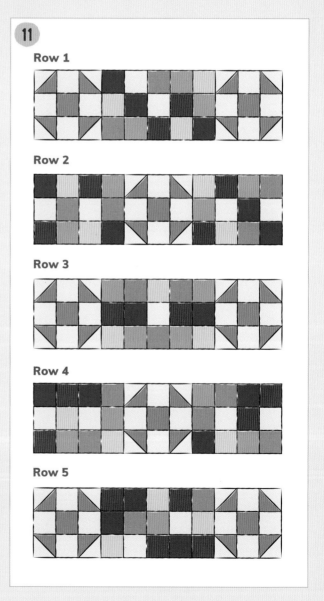

ADDING THE BORDERS

13 Trim the WOF border strips from Fabric H to 42in (106.75cm) in length by cutting off 1in (2.5cm) from each selvedge – the selvedges may shrink differently when you wash your patchwork, distorting the fabric, so it's best to trim them off.

14 Take two of the border strips and cut each into two pieces – one piece measuring 15in (40cm) and the other 27in (68.75cm).

15 Join a 42in (106.75cm) strip to a 15in (38cm) strip using a diagonal seam (see Steps 33–35 on page 117). Trim to 49½in (124.5cm). Repeat once more.

16 Join a 42in (106.75cm) strip to a 27in (68.75cm) strip using a diagonal seam. Trim to 60½in (153.75cm). Repeat once more.

17 Sew the longer border pieces to the left- and right-hand sides of the patchwork top, RS together, then press the seam allowances towards the borders. Join the shorter border pieces to the top and bottom edges of the patchwork top, again RS together, and then press the seam allowances towards the borders.

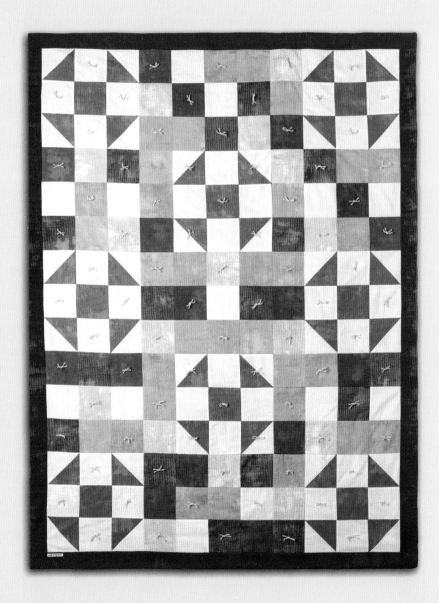

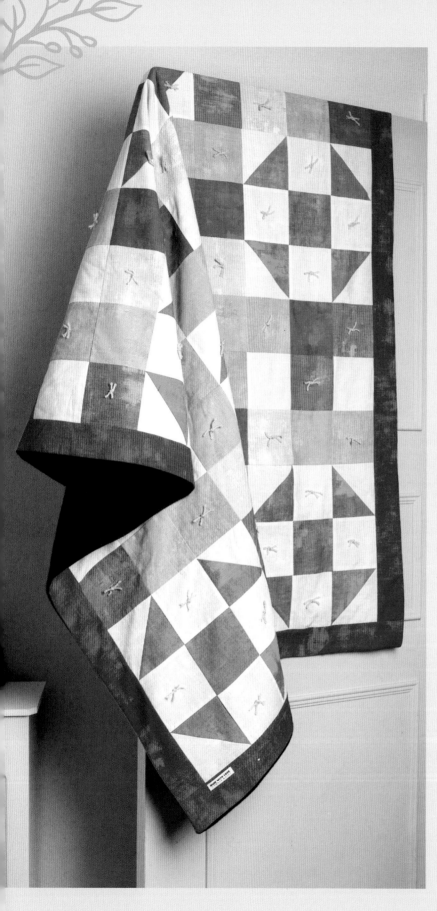

ASSEMBLING THE BLANKET

18 Lay the patchwork top over the fleece, RS together. Pin together, placing the curved safety pins at regular intervals approx. 5in (12.75cm) apart. Start pinning from the centre of the patchwork top and work outwards in each direction, stopping approx. 1–2in (2.5–5cm) from each edge. (See page 115 for more information.)

19 Once the layers are secure, sew all around the edge of the blanket with a ½in (1.25cm) seam allowance, leaving a 10in (25.5cm) gap at the centre-bottom edge for turning through.

20 Trim the seam allowances at the corners at a 45-degree angle to remove some of the bulk, being careful not to cut into the seam (see page 128).

21 Remove the pins then turn the blanket RS out through the gap. Poke out the corners using a point turner or another blunt-ended tool (like a chopstick, but nothing sharp like scissors!). Press the blanket from the patchwork top.

22 Sew the gap closed by hand with ladder stitch (see page 126).

TYING THE BLANKET

Note: We have chosen this finishing technique as it is time-efficient, and the ties add a nice textured effect to the blanket.

23 Referring to the photograph of the finished blanket on page 83, and leaving the squares in the corners of the blanket mark-free, mark the centre of every alternate square on the patchwork top. These will be the points where you'll add your ties.

24 Cut a 24in (61cm) length of thread. Thread it onto the needle and pull the ends to the same length for a doubled thread.

25 Select one of the marked squares at the centre of the blanket. Starting from the RS of the patchwork top, make a small stitch at the mark: take the threaded needle down through the mark and out the fleecy backing, then bring the needle back up to the patchwork top, close to your starting point.

26 Pull the thread through, leaving 2in (5cm) thread tails on top.

27 Trim your working thread (the needle end), leaving 2in (5cm) thread tails. Tie the thread tails into a double knot then trim them down to approx. ½in (1.25cm).

28 Working from the centre of the blanket outwards, tie the remaining marked squares in the same way. Please note that your ties may fluff up when you wash the blanket, but this just adds to its cozy charm!

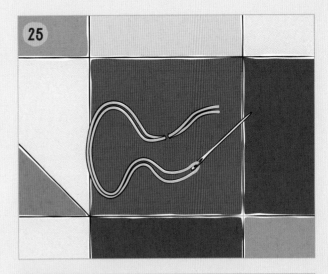

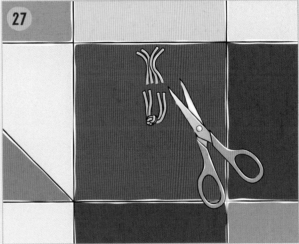

Behind the block names

The Shoo Fly quilt block dates from the 1850s and was found in many American patchworks. Well-known as a great block to help build confidence in piecing, it is part of the nine-patch block family with four Half Square Triangles at the corners. It has classic and timeless appeal and looks great in many combinations of fabric.

Symptom #8

BUTTER FINGERS

Who would have thought that menopause and clumsiness could go hand-in-hand? Well, they do! Oestrogen is thought to positively benefit fine motor skills, and so a drop in this hormone can affect your coordination and spatial awareness, leading to accidents.

To conquer slippery fingers, we've designed a slip-on apron with pockets that's perfect for protecting yourself against accidents, and for storing essentials too. The design is based on our best-selling pattern, the Hepworth Apron; we're delighted to include a new version of it in this book, knowing that hundreds of women have made the original design successfully already, and love to wear it.

The apron is designed to be extremely flattering and is suitable for all creative endeavours like baking, painting, gardening and sewing. It has a cross back and is comfortable to wear, with plenty of coverage and large patch pockets. When wearing it, just remember this golden rule: the only place where housework comes before needlework is in the dictionary!

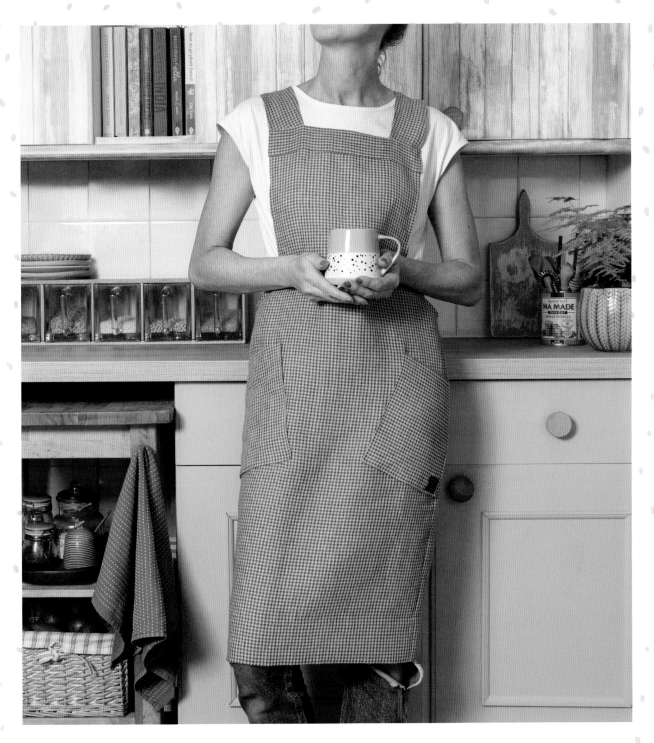

MAKER'S APRON

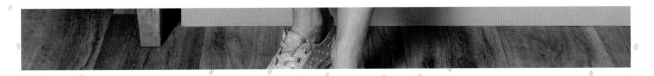

DIFFICULTY RATING

FINISHED SIZE

Will depend on size chosen; please refer to size chart below.

NOTES

- All seam allowances are ⅝in (1.5cm) unless stated otherwise.
- Sew using a stitch length of 3.0 unless stated otherwise.
- Always start and end with a backstitch when sewing a seam.
- Important: please trace all relevant templates; do not cut directly from the pattern sheet.

YOU WILL NEED

- Any hard-wearing, light- to medium-weight fabric will be perfect for your apron. A light denim would work well, and the apron hangs beautifully in washed linen. We've used European Linen Mini-Gingham in Hot Coral by Ray Stitch
- Seam gauge
- Maker's Apron templates A–D on Pattern Sheets A, B and C
- All-purpose or 40wt cotton thread

UK size (US size)	Size marked on template sheets	Bust measurement (circum.)	Hip measurement (circum.)	Width of Fabric (WOF) x length of fabric required
8–10 (4–6)	S–M	37⅜in (95cm)	39⅜in (100cm)	44in (11.75cm) WOF x 76in (193cm) 54in (138cm) WOF x 56in (142.5cm) 60in (152.5cm) WOF x 54in (137.5cm)
12–14 (8–10)	L–XL	39⅜in (100cm)	42½in (108cm)	44in (11.75cm) WOF x 76in (193cm) 54in (138cm) WOF x 56in (142.5cm) 60in (152.5cm) WOF x 54in (137.5cm)
16–18 (12–14)	XXL	42½in (108cm)	46in (117cm)	44in (11.75cm) WOF x 78in (198.5cm) 54in (138cm) WOF x 72in (183cm) 60in (152.5cm) WOF x 54in (137.5cm)
20–22 (16–18)	3XL	46in (117cm)	49⅝in (126cm)	44in (11.75cm) WOF x 78in (198.5cm) 54in (138cm) WOF x 72in (183cm) 60in (152.5cm) WOF x 72in (183cm)
24 (20)	4XL	49⅝in (126cm)	53⅛in (135cm)	44in (11.75cm) WOF x 83in (211cm) 54in (138cm) WOF x 76in (193cm) 60in (152.5cm) WOF x 72in (183cm)
26 (22)	5XL	53⅛in (135cm)	56¾in (144cm)	44in (11.75cm) WOF x 86in (218.5cm) 54in (138cm) WOF x 76in (193cm) 60in (152.5cm) WOF x 72in (183cm)
28 (24)	6XL	56¾in (144cm)	60⅝in (154cm)	44in (11.75cm) WOF x 86in (218.5cm) 54in (138cm) WOF x 76in (193cm) 60in (152.5cm) WOF x 72in (183cm)

CUTTING INSTRUCTIONS

Note: make sure to transfer all notch markings on the templates to your fabric (see page 140). Lay out all your pattern pieces on your fabric before cutting anything out, to ensure you make the most out of your fabric. If your fabric is directional, make sure your pattern pieces are orientated correctly.

- **Front (A)** – join the pattern as indicated then cut one on the fabric fold (see page 140)
- **Back (B)** – join the pattern as indicated then cut one pair from folded fabric
- **Front Band (C)** – cut one
- **Pockets (D)** – cut four

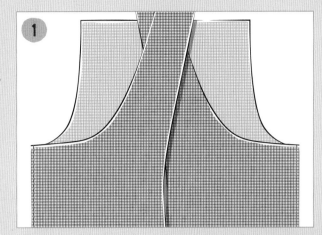

METHOD

JOINING THE FRONT & BACK PIECES

1 Place the back (B) pieces on top of the front (A) piece, *wrong sides* (WS) together and matching the notches. Pin at the side seams, then sew the side seams using a ¼in (5mm) seam allowance.

2 From the right side (RS), press the side seam allowances towards the front piece. Press again from the WS too, so that the seam and fabric lay flat.

3 Fold one back piece over the front piece, RS together, along the stitch line of the seam stitched in Step 1. The stitching should sit right on the edge of the fold. Press again. Secure with pins then stitch with a ⅜in (1cm) seam allowance, enclosing the raw edges of the fabric.

4 Press the seams towards the back piece. You have created a French seam!

5 Repeat Steps 3 and 4 with the other back piece.

6 Using small scissors, snip away a triangle at the top of both French seams. Start it ⅝in (1.5cm) below the raw edge and end it before reaching the row of stitching. This will reduce bulk in the hems around the armhole.

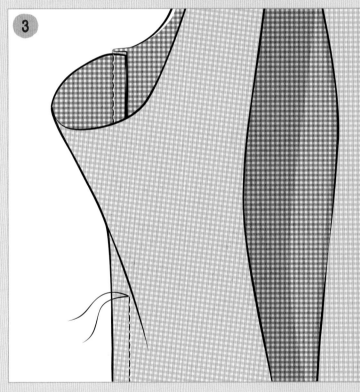

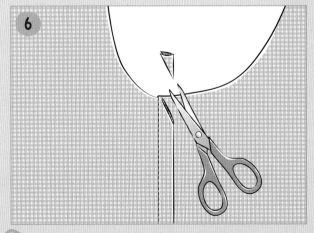

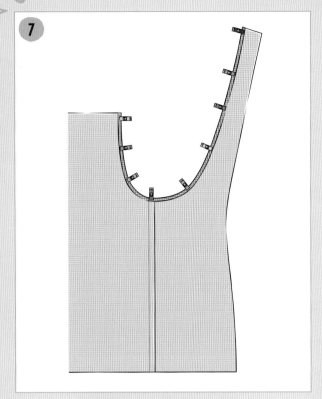

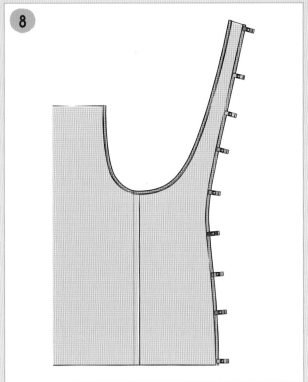

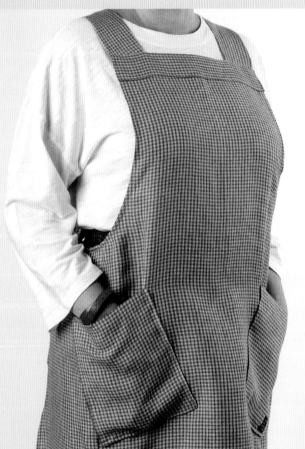

HEMMING THE ARMHOLE/STRAP EDGES

7 Along the armhole/strap edges (leave the top edge of the bib for now), turn under the fabric by ¼in (5mm), WS facing. Turn under the fabric by another ¼in (5mm) to create a double hem. Secure with pins or fabric clips. Edge-stitch close to the edge of the fold (see page 125). The trickiest part is going around the curve so take it slowly, especially over the French seams where the fabric is thicker.

HEMMING THE BACK EDGES

8 On the opposite side of the straps, down to the bottom of the apron back, turn under another double ¼in (5mm) hem, WS facing. Stitch in place as before. Press all hems.

POCKETS

9 If you wish, stitch a label onto the RS of one of the pocket (D) pieces. We added our label in the bottom right corner of the left pocket (refer to the photograph on page 87). If you're not stitching it into the seam (see page 143), make sure it's at least 1in (2.5cm) away from all edges, so it doesn't get caught in the seam allowance later.

10 Place two pocket pieces RS together and pin. Leaving a 2½in (6.25cm) gap along the centre-bottom edge, sew all around the pocket with a ⅜in (1cm) seam allowance. Backstitch at the beginning and end of the seam line, and pivot at the corners to make these as sharp as possible when you turn the pockets RS out later (see pages 124 and 127). Clip across the corners of the seam allowances at a 45-degree angle (see page 128), to reduce bulk in these parts of the seam. Repeat to make the second pocket.

11 Turn each pocket RS out through the gap. Poke out the corners using a point turner or another blunt-ended tool (like a chopstick, but nothing sharp like scissors!). Press the pockets, turning the raw edges of the gap towards the inside to neaten.

12 Pin or clip the straps to the bib of the apron front temporarily – make sure to cross the straps and to pin the ends of the strap ½in (1.25cm) below the raw edges of the bib. Try on the apron, then pin the pockets into a position that is comfortable for you; your hands should touch the bottom of the pockets when they are slipped inside them – the pocket placement lines on template A is where we think they should be about right. Take off the apron, unpin the straps then baste/tack the pockets in place.

13 Sew the pockets in place around the side and bottom edges with top-stitching (see page 125), backstitching at the ends of the stitching to give the pocket opening some strength. The top-stitching will close up the turning gap in each pocket too.

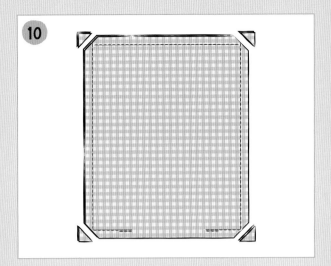

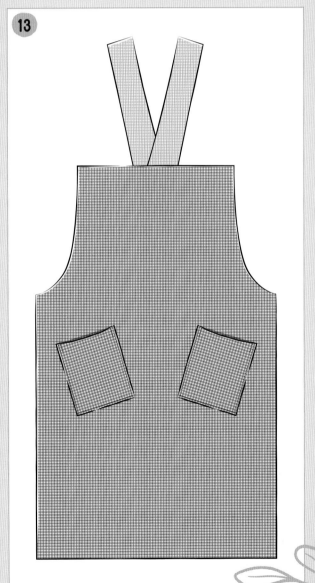

ATTACHING THE STRAPS & FRONT BAND

14 Turn under and press a ⅜in (1cm) hem along the bottom edge of the front band (C) piece, WS together. Next turn under and press a ⅝in (1.5cm) hem on both short ends of the front band, again WS together. Lay the front band on top of the apron bib to ensure that they are the same width as each other. Set the front band aside.

15 Lay the apron so the WS is facing up. Fold the back pieces over the apron front, so WS are together. Cross the straps and align the unfinished top edges of the straps to the top of the bib at each end, as shown. Secure them in place with a row of basting/tacking stitches, ¼in (5mm) below the raw edge.

16 Lay the RS of the front band over the WS of the apron bib, matching the raw edges. The straps should be sandwiched between the two layers. Pin in place, then stitch along the top of the bib with a ½in (1.25cm) seam allowance. Clip across the corners at a 45-degree angle, within the seam allowance (see page 128). Press the seam allowance away from the bib.

17 Fold the front band over to the RS of the apron and press, so the stitching sits right on the edge of the fold. Secure the three remaining edges temporarily with pins or basting/tacking stitches, then edge-stitch all around the front band (see page 125). Take care not to stitch into the back section of the apron when you do this!

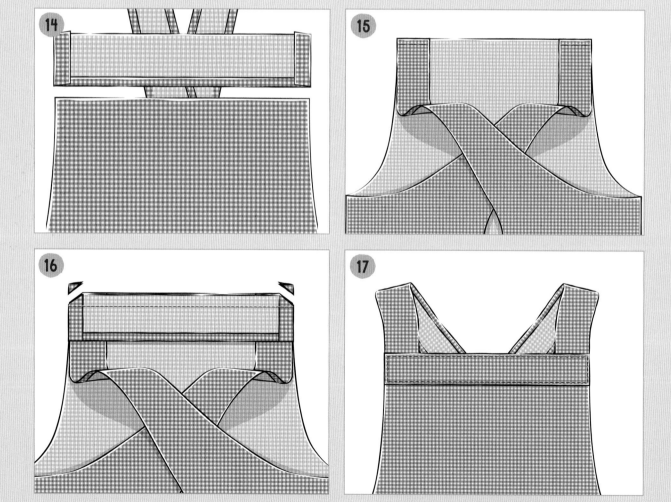

SEWING THE HEM

18 Turn under the bottom edge of the apron by ½in (1.25cm), WS together, then fold the fabric again by 3in (7.5cm). Stitch in place along the hem's fold. You can leave the free ends open, or close the gaps by machine or hand with ladder stitch (see page 126).

19 Trim all threads and give the apron a good press. A damp pressing cloth will help to remove the crease down the centre front of the apron and to protect the fabric.

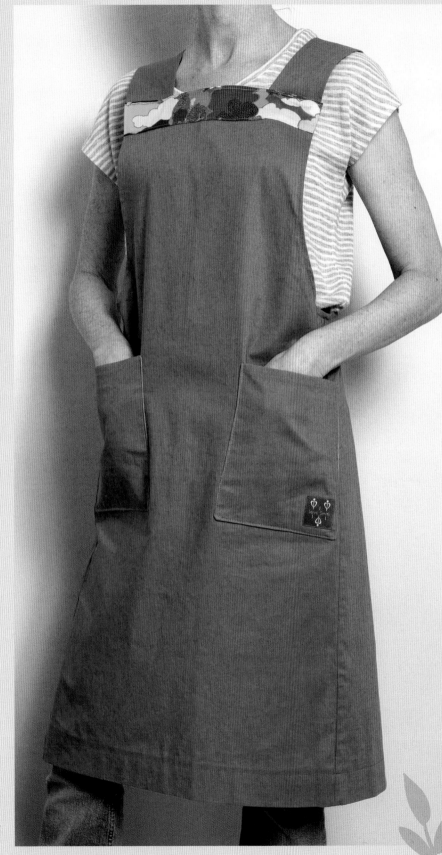

A variation, this time using washed linen for the apron front and back and pockets, and our favourite Prospect Road Liberty™ fabric for the front band.

Symptom #9
HOT FLASHES

Hot flashes are the most common symptom of the menopausal transition. Experienced at any time of the day, sudden warmth is felt across the upper body, often combined with increased heart rate and perspiration. While their frequency and intensity differ among women, they do cause real discomfort and can stick around for an average of 7 to 10 years.

So, let our super stylish (and simple to construct) Cool-down Cover-up ease the discomfort of unwanted heat and fill you with pride as you flaunt your dressmaking ability!

This loose-fitting jacket is a forgiving pattern for those new to sewing their own clothes, as there are no zips, buttons or other fastenings to contend with. It is also very flattering for changes in body shape since it has a gentle silhouette, and the cover-up easily coordinates with numerous other items of clothing including dresses, trousers, T-shirts and even beachwear.

We love how our friend, Alison Lewis from the Liberty™ haberdashery department, models this jacket on the following pages with effortless style.

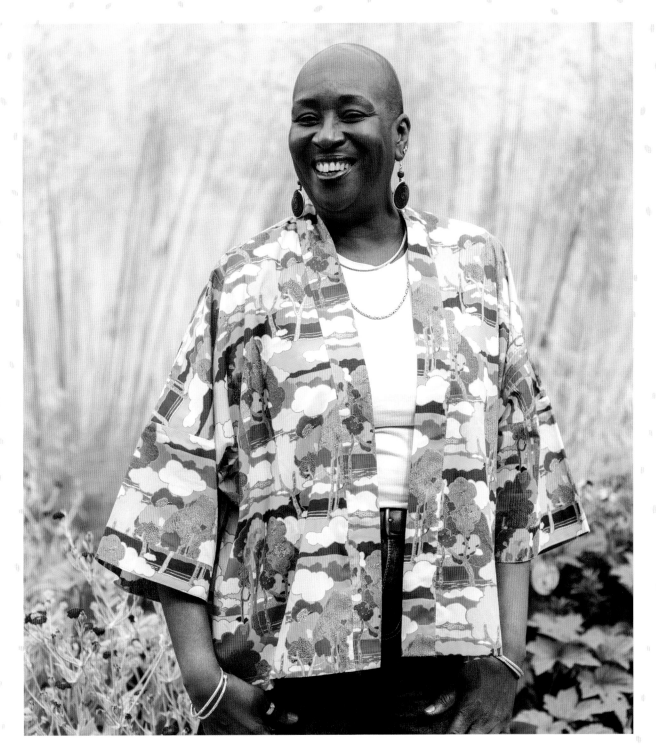

COOL-DOWN COVER-UP

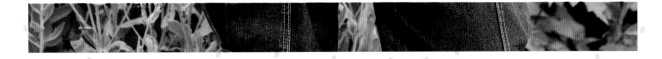

DIFFICULTY RATING

FINISHED SIZE

Will depend on size chosen; please refer to the size chart opposite.

NOTES

- All seam allowances are ⅝in (1.5cm) unless stated otherwise.
- Sew using a stitch length of 3.0.
- Always start and end with a backstitch when sewing a seam.
- Important: please trace all relevant templates; do not cut directly from the pattern sheet.

YOU WILL NEED

- Light- to medium-weight woven fabric, in the quantity detailed in the size chart opposite – we recommend cotton lawn as this drapes beautifully and feels floaty, and we've used Prospect Road in Tana Lawn™ by Liberty™
- Thread to match fabric – use 50wt for cotton lawn or 40wt for heavier cottons
- Machine needle in size 70/10 for cotton lawn or 80/12 for heavier cottons
- Seam gauge
- Cool-down Cover-up templates A–E on Pattern Sheets D, E and F

CUTTING INSTRUCTIONS

Note: make sure to transfer all notch markings on the templates to your fabric (see page 140). Lay out all your pattern pieces on your fabric before cutting anything out, to ensure you make the most out of your fabric. If your fabric is directional, make sure your pattern pieces are orientated correctly.

- **Back (A)** – cut one on fabric fold (see page 140)
- **Front (B)** – cut once from folded fabric, so you cut a symmetrical pair of fronts
- **Sleeve (C)** – cut two
- **Cuff (D)** – cut two
- **Neckband/collar (E)** – cut two, with the 'joining end' at the top

> "Success is liking yourself, liking what you do, and liking how you do it."
>
> MAYA ANGELOU

UK size (US size)	Size marked on template sheets	Bust measurement (circum.)	Hip measurement (circum.)	Width of Fabric (WOF) x length of fabric required
8–10 (4–6)	S–M	37⅜in (95cm)	39⅜in (100cm)	44in (11.75cm) WOF x 80in (203.5cm) 54in (138cm) WOF x 60in (152.5cm) 60in (152.5cm) WOF x 48in (122cm)
12–14 (8–10)	L–XL	39⅜in (100cm)	42½in (108cm)	44in (11.75cm) WOF x 81in (193cm) 54in (138cm) WOF x 61in (142.5cm) 60in (152.5cm) WOF x 50in (137.5cm)
16–18 (12–14)	XXL	42½in (108cm)	46in (117cm)	44in (11.75cm) WOF x 82in (208.5cm) 54in (138cm) WOF x 62in (157.5cm) 60in (152.5cm) WOF x 62in (157.5cm)
20–22 (16–18)	3XL	46in (117cm)	49⅝in (126cm)	44in (11.75cm) WOF x 84in (213.5cm) 54in (138cm) WOF x 71in (180.5cm) 60in (152.5cm) WOF x 64in (162.5cm)
24 (20)	4XL	49⅝in (126cm)	53⅛in (135cm)	44in (11.75cm) WOF x 96in (244cm) 54in (138cm) WOF x 74in (188cm) 60in (152.5cm) WOF x 64in (162.5cm)
26 (22)	5XL	53⅛in (135cm)	56¾in (144cm)	44in (11.75cm) WOF x 97in (246.5cm) 54in (138cm) WOF x 74in (188cm) 60in (152.5cm) WOF x 74in (188cm)
28 (24)	6XL	56¾in (144cm)	60⅝in (154cm)	44in (11.75cm) WOF x 98in (249cm) 54in (138cm) WOF x 76in (193cm) 60in (152.5cm) WOF x 76in (193cm)

Getting busy with it

A busy pattern, like the one we've used, or a general all-over pattern is often the best choice for beginners. It obscures the seams and top-stitching, and means mistakes are easily hidden! A fabric with a very distinct repeating motif will require pattern matching, so you might want to try this once you've had plenty of practice!

METHOD

JOINING THE FRONT & BACK PIECES

1 Place the front (B) pieces on top of the back (A) piece, *wrong sides* (WS) together and matching the notches. Pin at the shoulder seams, then sew using a ¼in (5mm) seam allowance.

2 Open out the fabrics flat, so both right sides (RS) of the stitched front and back are facing up. From the RS, press the seam allowance towards the back piece. Press again from the WS too, so that the seam and fabric lie flat.

3 Fold the front and back fabrics RS together, along the stitch line of the seam stitched in Step 1; the stitching should sit right on the edge of the fold. Press again. Secure with pins then stitch with a ⅜in (1cm) seam allowance, enclosing the raw edges of the fabric.

4 Press the seams towards the back piece. You have created French seams!

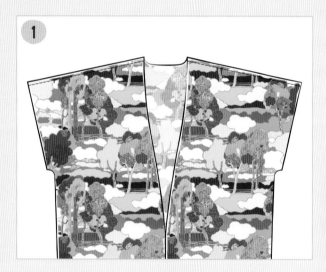

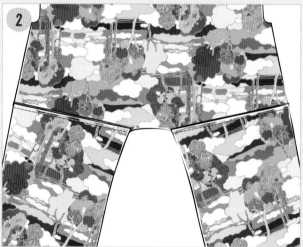

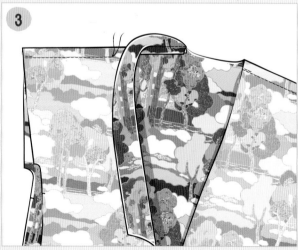

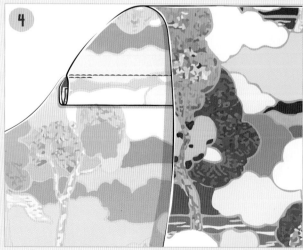

ADDING THE CUFFS TO THE SLEEVE

5 Fold one cuff (D) piece in half WS together, matching the notches. Press. Unfold; you should have a lengthwise crease along the middle.

6 Turn under the bottom edge of the cuff piece by ⅝in (1.5cm), WS together. Press.

7 Centre the D piece along the bottom edge of one sleeve (C) piece, RS together, matching the raw edges and notches, and with the fold from Step 5 pointing up towards the sleeve. Pin then sew along the raw edges.

8 Press the seam allowance towards the cuff piece from the WS. Flip over the joined pieces then press from the RS.

9 Fold the cuff piece over the bottom raw edge of the sleeve, until the crease line pressed in Step 5 aligns with the bottom edge, and the turned-under bottom edge of the cuff made in Step 6 is on the WS of the sleeve, just covering the stitch line. Pin or baste/tack in place.

10 Edge-stitch along both top and bottom seams (see page 125).

11 Repeat Steps 5–10 with the remaining cuff and sleeve pieces.

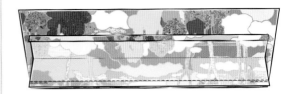

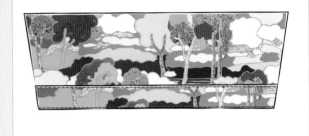

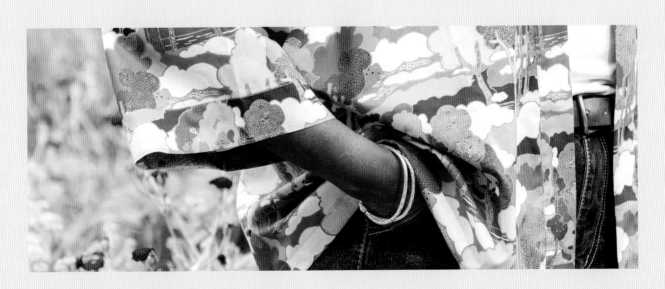

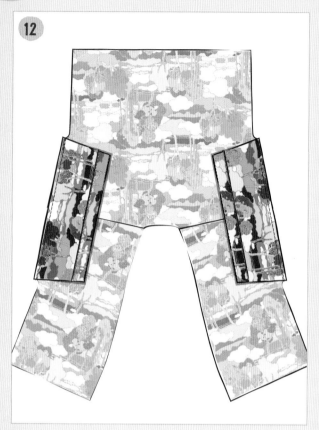

ATTACHING THE SLEEVES

12 Open out the front/back pieces then centre the sleeves over the shoulder seams, WS together, raw edges matching, and aligning the centre notch of each sleeve with a shoulder seam. Pin then sew with a ¼in (5mm) seam allowance.

13 Press the seam allowances towards the front/back pieces, first from the RS then the WS.

14 Turn the seams into French seams: fold one sleeve towards the front/back pieces, RS together and along the stitch line from the seam stitched in Step 12. The stitching should sit right on the edge of the fold. Press, secure with pins then sew along this edge with a ⅜in (1cm) seam allowance, enclosing the raw edge. Press the seam towards the sleeve. Repeat to finish the French seam on the other sleeve.

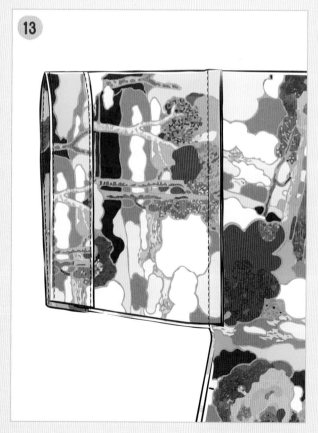

ADDING THE NECKBAND/COLLAR

15 Sew the short joining end of one neckband/collar (E) piece to the short joining end of the other neckband/collar piece, RS together, to create one long strip. Press the seam allowance open. If your fabric is directional, join with the top of the design at the seam for both neckband/collar pieces.

16 Press the strip in half along its length, WS together and matching the notches. Unfold; you should have a lengthwise crease along the middle.

17 Turn under one long edge by ⅝in (1.5cm), WS together, then press.

18 Aligning the seam of the neckband/collar piece with the back neckline (piece A), pin the neckband/collar around the neckline and front opening of the front/back pieces, RS together, matching raw edges and aligning the notches. Sew in place.

19 Notch the curve of the neckline, taking care not to cut into the stitching (see page 128).

20 Press the seam allowance towards the neckband/collar from the WS (see the tip below for help with this). Flip over the garment then press from the RS.

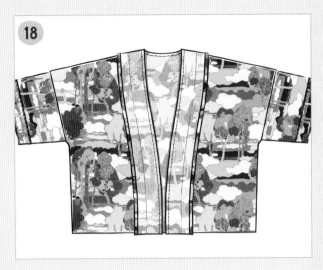

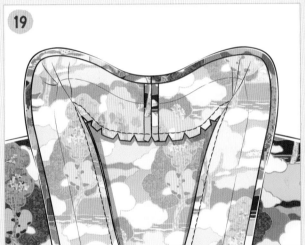

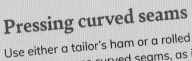

Pressing curved seams

Use either a tailor's ham or a rolled up towel to press curved seams, as it will help you get around the curve.

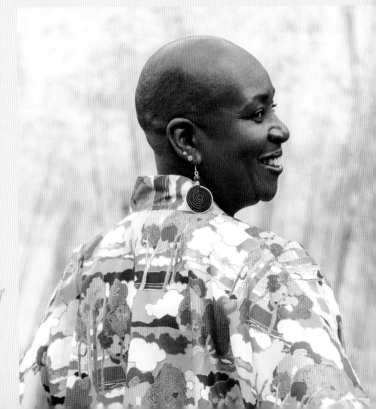

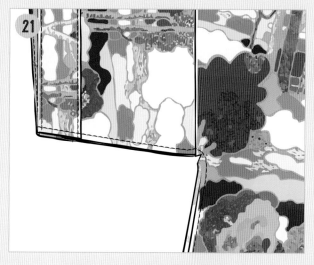

JOINING THE SIDE SEAMS

21 Turn the garment RS out, so WS are together. Match the notches at the side seams and pin. Sew with a ¼in (5mm) seam allowance from the cuff edge, around the under arm curve to the bottom edge. Clip the corner at the underarm, within the seam allowance, to reduce bulk in this part of the seam (see page 128).

22 Press the seam allowance towards the back section from the RS, then flip the garment and press the seam allowance once more from the WS.

23 Turn the side seams into French seams: turn the garment WS out, so RS are together. Press the side seam allowances towards the back once more; the stitching should sit right on the edge of the fold. Secure with pins then stitch with a ⅜in (1cm) seam allowance, enclosing the raw edge. Press towards the back piece.

HEMMING THE BOTTOM EDGE

24 Fold over the whole bottom edge of the garment by 1in (2.5cm), WS together. Press.

25 Fold the corners of the front opening into a triangle, creating a 45-degree angle on both sides.

26 Fold over the hem once more, again by 1in (2.5cm), to make a double hem (see page 128).

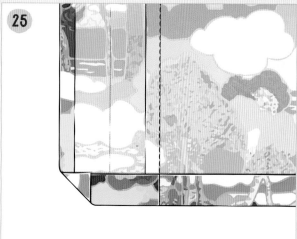

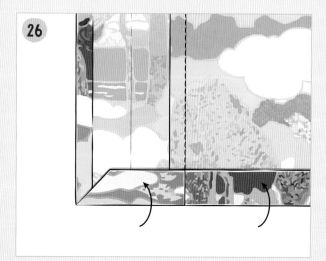

27 With WS together, fold the neckband/collar along the central crease pressed in Step 16. Pin or clip in place, so all the seam allowances are enclosed.

28 From the RS, sew the bottom hem in place with a ¾in (2cm) seam allowance, starting from the seam of the band on one front opening and finishing at the seam of the band on the opposite front opening. Press.

29 Baste/tack the loose, folded edge of the neckband/collar in place over the seam where it was joined in Step 18. Sew in place with edge-stitching (see page 125). Press the seam allowance from the WS.

30 Trim all threads and then give the cover-up a good press. Wear it with pride!

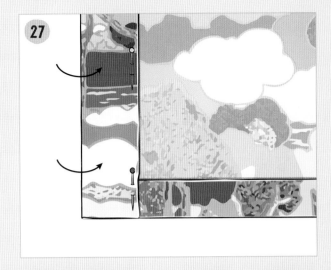

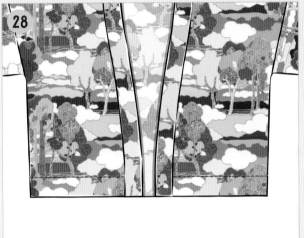

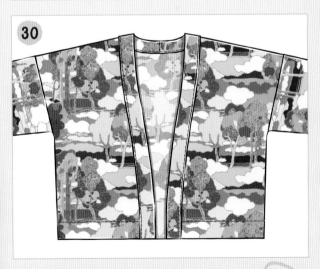

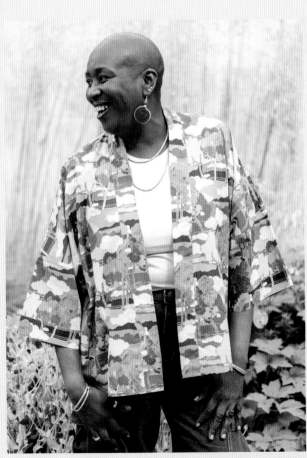

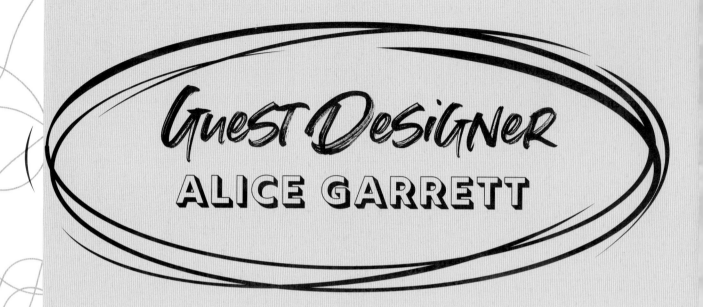

GUEST DESIGNER
ALICE GARRETT

Alice Garrett is an entrepreneurial maker and business owner with a shared passion for one of our favourite fabric manufacturers in the world – Liberty™. We love browsing her online shop, Alice Caroline, which presents a stunning array of Liberty™ fabrics, many of which can be bought in small pieces, making them affordable for the projects in this book. We promise that you will be spoilt for choice!

Alice designs beautiful quilts and sewing projects for all abilities, runs an award-winning company, and also founded the incredible Quilt SOS project, which co-ordinates the sewing and donating of quilts to women and children in need. It's always a joy to bump into Alice and her team at the Festival of Quilts in Birmingham, UK, and to compare notes on our handmade outfits before buying some lovely, light-weight Tana Lawn™ to sew up!

Jenni & Kay x

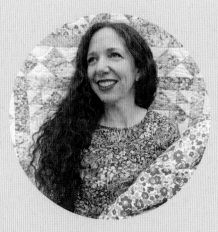

A Few Words From Alice:

'I started Alice Caroline because I am passionate about helping people connect with their creativity, and bringing people together through a shared love of beautiful fabrics and sewing. I learned to sew from my grandmother, and recognize how sewing can create bonds across potential generational gaps. I love meeting three generations of sewers together at sewing festivals.

Crafting and sewing can be a way for people, especially those who may have always prioritized others, to tune into their own needs and explore new creative avenues. Going through the menopause presents that opportunity for change, even though it can be rocky and we can't see the way through sometimes. I'm finding it so essential to talk to friends about various symptoms, and discovering that we're all in the same boat in some way or another is comforting! I am mindful that previous generations didn't really have this opportunity to speak so openly and yet they made it through, one stitch at a time.'

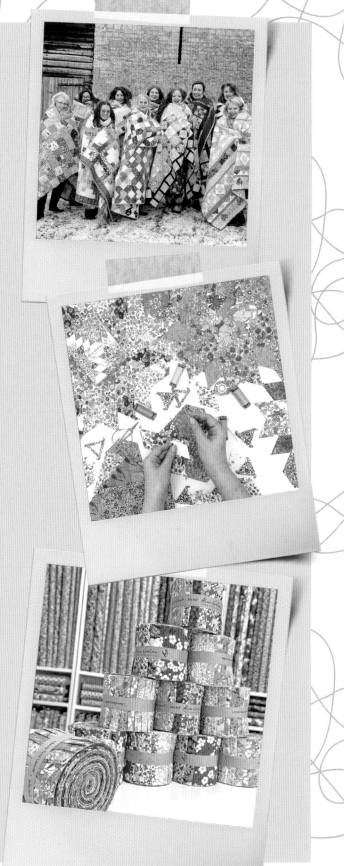

Symptom #10

NIGHT SWEATS

Hormonal changes in menopause affect your brain's ability to regulate body temperature and sadly the symptom of night sweats can be very uncomfortable and disruptive. Women can feel intensely hot on most parts of their body, and can sweat profusely to try to cool their core temperature.

It is important to sleep beneath natural fibres such as cotton as they allow moisture to evaporate through the fabric, helping you stay cooler while you sleep and wake up feeling fresher.

Therefore, our quilt is the perfect project both to take care of yourself and add real style and homemade charm to your bedroom. Stitched in 100% cotton or cotton lawn, it feels beautifully soft and soothing against your skin, setting the intention for a good night's sleep. You could use this as a cooler substitute to your normal duvet.

Quilts can seem daunting to make, but once finished they become both comfort blankets and heirlooms. So, we encourage you all to give this project a go!

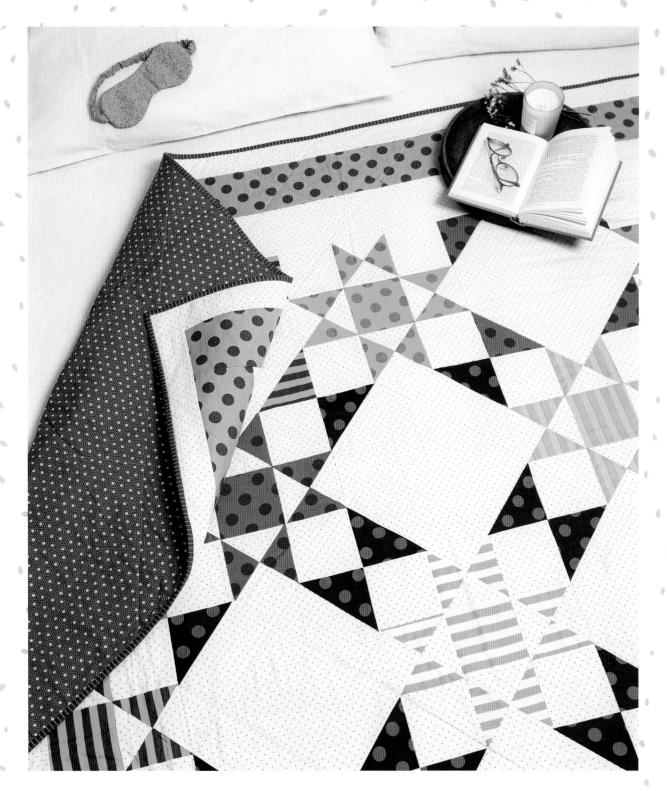

KEEP COOL QUILT

DIFFICULTY RATING

FINISHED SIZE

Finished quilt: 80in (203.25cm) square

Unfinished block size: 12½in (31.75cm) square

Finished block size: 12in (30.5cm) square

YOU WILL NEED

Fabrics (we've used the True Colours collection by Tula Pink for Free Spirit Fabrics; the specific colours are detailed in brackets):

- Fabric A (Tiny Dots in Cosmic/pink-on-white) – one 4½yd x WOF (162 x 44in/460 x 112cm) for the background and Borders 1 and 3
- Fabric B (Pom Poms in Foxglove/purple-pink polka dot) – one Fat Quarter (22 x 18in/56 x 45.75cm) for the Snowball blocks
- Fabric C (Pom Poms in Peony/pink-red polka dot) – one Fat Quarter (22 x 18in/56 x 45.75cm) for the Ohio Star and Snowball blocks
- Fabric D (Pom Poms in Lupine/blue-red polka dot) – one Fat Quarter (22 x 18in/56 x 45.75cm) for the Ohio Star and Snowball blocks
- Fabric E (Pom Poms in Agave/mint-brown polka dot) – one Fat Quarter (22 x 18in/56 x 45.75cm) for the Ohio Star and Snowball blocks
- Fabric F (Tent Stripe in Iris/purple-mint stripe) – one Fat Quarter (22 x 18in/56 x 45.75cm) for the Ohio Star and Snowball blocks
- Fabric G (Tent Stripe in Myrtle/blue-lime stripe) – one Fat Quarter (22 x 18in/56 x 45.75cm) for the Ohio Star and Snowball blocks

NOTES

- All seam allowances are ¼in (5mm) unless stated otherwise.
- Sew all patchwork using a stitch length of 2.2.
- Always press from the back first then turn over and press again from the front.
- The width-of-fabric (WOF) measurements assume you are cutting from a bolt measuring 44in (112cm) wide; check the width of the bolt when purchasing your own fabric.
- Refer to pages 130 and 131 for information on cutting your patchwork pieces.

- Fabric H (Tent Stripe in Peony/pink-red stripe) – one Fat Quarter (22 x 18in/56 x 45.75cm) for the Ohio Star and Snowball blocks
- Fabric I (Tent Stripe in Begonia/orange-cream stripe) – one Fat Quarter (22 x 18in/56 x 45.75cm) for the Ohio Star and Snowball blocks
- Fabric J (Pom Poms in Lupine/blue-red polkadot) – one 1yd x WOF (36 x 44in/91.5 x 112cm), for the Border 2
- Fabric K (Tiny Stripes in Astor/purple-pink thin stripe) – one ¾yd x WOF (27 x 44in/70 x 112cm), for the quilt binding
- Fabric L (Hexy in Thistle/purple-mint hexagon spot) – one 5yd x WOF (180 x 44in/460 x 112cm), for the quilt backing

Everything else:

- One 88in (2.25m) square of batting/wadding
- Square quilting ruler, minimum 4½ x 4½in (11.5 x 11.5cm)
- Basting/tacking tools of your choice (see page 115)
- Hera marker
- Walking (even-/dual-feed) foot
- 50wt cotton thread for piecing and quilting

CUTTING INSTRUCTIONS

From Fabric A:

- Twelve 12½in (31.75cm) squares, for the Snowball block centres
- Twenty-six 5½in (14cm) squares
- Fifty-two 4½in (11.5cm) squares
- Eight 4½in (11.5cm) x WOF strips, for Border 1
- Eight 2½in (6.25cm) x WOF strips, for Border 3

From Fabric B (this will yield four Snowball blocks):

- Sixteen 4½in (11.5cm) squares

Each from Fabrics C–H (this will yield two Ohio Stars blocks and one Snowball block from each fabric; twelve Ohio Stars blocks and six Snowball blocks in total):

- Four 5½in (14cm) squares
- Six 4½in (11.5cm) squares

From Fabric I (this will yield one Ohio Star block and two Snowball blocks):

- Two 5½in (14cm) squares
- Nine 4½in (11.5cm) squares

From Fabric J:

- Eight 4½in (11.5cm) x WOF strips

From Fabric K:

- Eight 2¼in (5.75cm) x WOF strips

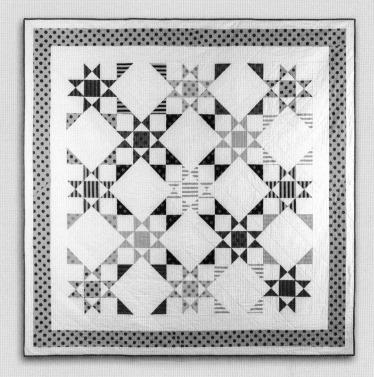

Behind the Ohio Star and Hourglass blocks names

The Ohio Star block is steeped in history and has been around since the early 1800s. It was popular among the pioneer quilters in America, and is a great introduction to Quarter Square Triangles (also known as the Hourglass block). As you stitch, imagine a beautiful starry sky similar to those that the pioneers would have been travelling beneath to start a new life.

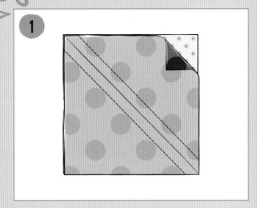

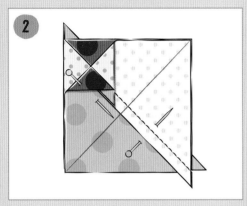

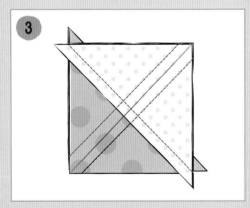

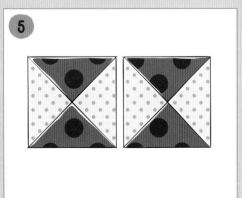

METHOD

MAKING THE HOURGLASS BLOCKS

1 We will be using the two-at-a-time method to make Half Square Triangles (HSTs). Draw a diagonal line on the wrong side (WS) of one 5½in (14cm) Fabric C square. Place this square over a 5½in (14cm) Fabric A square, right sides (RS) facing, and pin together. Sew a ¼in (5mm) away from each side of the drawn line, as shown. Cut along the drawn line to create two HSTs. Press the seam allowances towards the darker fabric.

2 Place the two HSTs RS together, making sure that the matching fabrics are not facing each other, and the seams align and nest. The illustration shows a corner of the top fabric folded back to demonstrate how they nest. Draw a diagonal line along the top HST, making it perpendicular to the seam.

3 Sew a ¼in (5mm) away from each side of the drawn line, as shown.

4 Cut along the drawn line and press the seams to one side to make two Hourglass blocks.

5 Trim the blocks down to 4½in (11.5cm) square using a rotary cutter and square quilting ruler: line up the 2¼in (5.75cm) marks (both horizontal and vertical) on the ruler with the point where all four triangles meet in the centre of the block. At the top and right-hand sides, trim away any excess you see extending beyond the ruler. Rotate the block 180 degrees. Trim the block again, this time lining up the ruler along the bottom and left-hand edges on the 4½in (11.5cm) lines. Trim away any excess you see on the top and right-hand sides.

6 Repeat Steps 1–5 with the remaining 5½in (14cm) squares cut from Fabrics B–I, pairing each of the 5½in (14cm) squares with a 5½in (14cm) Fabric A square, creating a total of fifty-two Hourglass Blocks.

ASSEMBLING THE OHIO STAR BLOCKS

7 Sew a 4½in (11.5cm) Fabric A square to the left-hand side of one Fabric C Hourglass block, RS together and with the Hourglass block on its side. Press the seam allowance towards the Fabric A square.

8 Sew another 4½in (11.5cm) Fabric A square to the right-hand side of the unit created in Step 7. Press the seam allowance towards the Fabric A square.

9 Repeat Steps 7 and 8 to make an identical unit of three squares.

10 Using the same fabrics and referring to the illustration for the orientation of the Hourglass blocks, sew an Hourglass block to either side of a 4½in (11.5cm) Fabric C square, RS together. Press the seam allowances towards the centre square.

11 Arrange the three units, so that the row made in Step 10 is in between the units made in Steps 7–9. Sew the three rows RS together, pinning at the seams beforehand to align them accurately. Press the seam allowances towards the centre row.

12 Repeat Steps 7–11 with the forty-eight remaining Hourglass blocks, forty-eight 4½in (11.5cm) Fabric A squares, and the 4½in (11.5cm) squares cut from Fabrics B–I (one each from Fabrics C and I, and two each from the rest). You will have thirteen Ohio Star blocks in total, in seven different colourways.

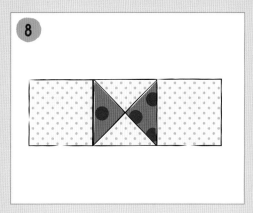

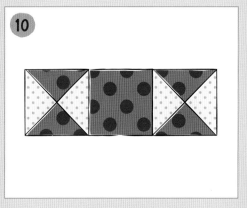

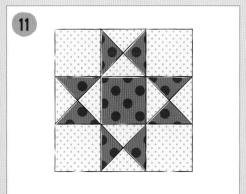

Working with stripes

If you are using striped fabric like we have, don't worry about its direction in Step 2 – you will automatically end up with one Hourglass block with vertical stripes and one with horizontal stripes. If you wish, you can keep the orientation of the stripes consistent within each Ohio Star block, including the centre square. You can then position the block either horizontally or vertically within the quilt.

MAKING THE SNOWBALL BLOCKS

13 Draw a diagonal line on the WS of four 4½in (11.5cm) Fabric C squares. With RS facing, place a square in each corner of one 12½in (31.75cm) Fabric A square, matching the outer raw edges, and pin. The diagonal lines of the top two squares should point from the sides to the centre-top edge, and the diagonal lines of the bottom two squares should point from the sides to the centre-bottom edge.

14 Sew along the drawn line of each patterned square.

15 Trim away the corner 'triangles', ¼in (5mm) away from the sewn line with a rotary cutter and ruler, as shown. Fold back the corner squares and press the seam allowances flat from both sides.

16 Repeat Steps 13–15 with the remaining eleven 12½in (31.75cm) Fabric A squares and forty-four 4½in (11.5cm) squares in Fabrics B–E. You will have twelve Snowball blocks in total, in seven different colourways.

ASSEMBLING THE QUILT TOP

17 Lay out the blocks in five rows of five, referring to the photograph of the finished quilt on page 109 and the illustration opposite to decide placement of the different fabrics, and the orientation of the blocks (particularly if you have used stripes).

18 When you're happy with the arrangement, first sew the five blocks in each row RS together, matching the seams. Press the seam allowances for each row in alternate directions: press the seam allowances in the top row to the right, the seam allowances in the second row to the left, the seam allowances in the third row to the right, and so on.

19 Join the rows RS together, then press these new seam allowances downwards.

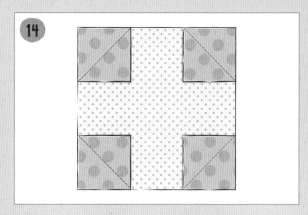

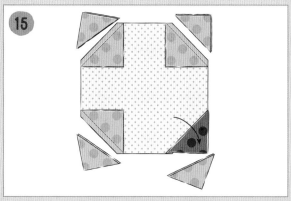

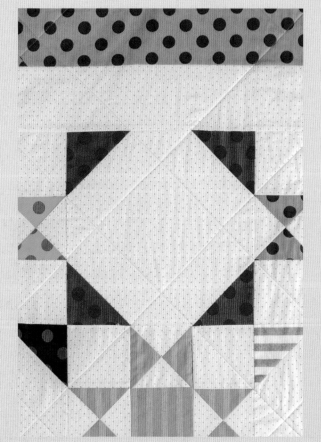

MAKING THE BORDER STRIPS

20 Trim the WOF strips to 42in (106.75cm) in length by cutting off 1in (2.5cm) from each selvedge – the selvedges may shrink differently when you wash your patchwork, distorting the fabric, so it's best to trim them off.

21 Make up **Border 1:**

– Sew two 4½in (11.5cm) x 42in (106.75cm) Fabric A strips RS together, using a diagonal seam (see Steps 33–35 on page 117 for more information). Trim to 60½in (153.75cm). Repeat to make another border strip.

– Sew two 4½in (11.5cm) x 42in (106.75cm) Fabric A strips RS together, using a diagonal seam. Trim to 68½in (174cm). Repeat to make another border strip.

22 Make up **Border 2:**

– Sew two 4½in (11.5cm) x 42in (106.75cm) Fabric J strips RS together, using a diagonal seam. Trim to 68½in (174cm). Repeat to make another border strip.

– Sew two 4½in (11.5cm) x 42in (106.75cm) Fabric J strips RS together, using a diagonal seam. Trim to 76½in (194.25cm). Repeat to make another border strip.

23 Make up **Border 3:**

– Sew two 2½in (6.25cm) x 42in (106.75cm) Fabric A strips RS together, using a diagonal seam. Trim to 76½in (194.25cm). Repeat to make another border strip.

– Sew two 2½in (6.25cm) x 42in (106.75cm) Fabric A strips RS together, using a diagonal seam. Trim to 80½in (204.5cm). Repeat to make another border strip.

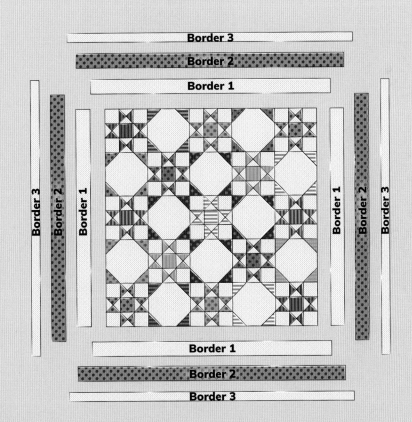

ADDING BORDERS TO THE QUILT TOP

24 Start with the Border 1 pieces. Pin the shorter borders to the left- and right-hand sides of the quilt top, RS together and raw edges matching, and pinning at regular intervals. Sew in place then press the seam allowances towards the borders. Pin and sew the longer borders to the quilt in the same way, this time along the top and bottom edges.

25 Repeat Step 24 with the Border 2 pieces, followed by the Border 3 pieces.

MAKING THE QUILT SANDWICH & PREPPING FOR QUILTING

26 Cut the backing fabric into two equal 2½yd (230cm) x WOF pieces and sew RS together along the longest edges using a 1in (2.5cm) seam allowance. Press the seam allowance to one side.

27 Lay the backing RS down then centre the batting/wadding on top. (**Note:** the batting/wadding won't be the same size as the backing, but that's fine.) Centre the quilt top over the two layers, RS facing up. The backing and batting/wadding will be bigger than the quilt top; this is correct. Keep the layers straight so that the grain of the backing fabric and the grain of the quilt top are aligned (see pages 122 and 123).

28 Baste/tack the three layers of the quilt sandwich together using your preferred basting/tacking method – see the info box opposite for more details.

QUILTING

29 Using either hand or machine quilting (see pages 134–137 for more details), quilt as desired or refer to the pattern in the diagram below.

Tips:

– We recommend marking the quilt with a hera marker before quilting, especially if you will be quilting lines, so you have some guidelines to follow.

– If you are quilting by hand you will need your chosen thread (see page 133 for suggestions), a quilting needle in the size that's suitable for your thread, and a thimble. An optional extra is a quilters' hoop.

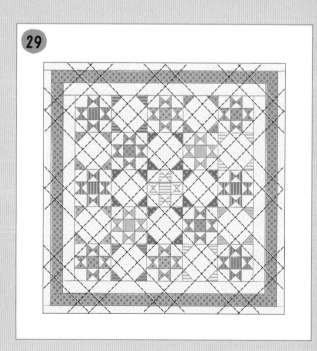

BASTING/TACKING A QUILT

Basting/tacking is when you use a temporary method of securing the three layers of the 'quilt sandwich' together. A quilt sandwich is made up of a backing fabric on the bottom (RS facing down), the batting/wadding in the middle, and quilt top on top (RS facing up). Always ensure that the batting/wadding and backing are larger than the quilt top by at least 2in (5cm) on all sides; this is because sometimes the quilt top can 'grow' when flattened out and quilted. The excess is trimmed away after the quilting stage.

There are various methods of basting/tacking your quilt:

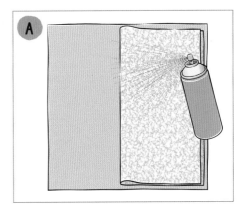

- **Spray basting (A)** uses a temporary spray adhesive that then can be washed out. This is the fastest method, but not the most cost effective. Follow the instructions on the can to make sure you apply and set the adhesive correctly.

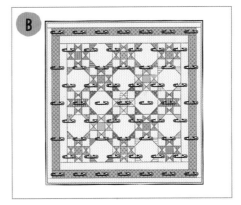

- **Pin basting (B)** uses safety pins or specially made curved safety pins. Once your sandwich layers are made up, place the safety pins in rows across the quilt top at approx. 5in (12.75cm) intervals, starting from the centre of the quilt and working outwards. Consider the surface you are pinning your quilt on, and be careful not to scratch it when putting the pins in place – it may not be a good idea to pin on your best dining table!

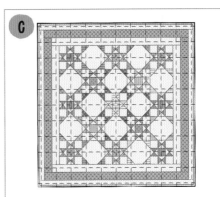

- **Thread basting (C)** is done by hand. We recommend using 100% cotton thread as it will not snag your quilt top when removed. Starting from the centre of the quilt and working outwards, stitch large running stitches across the quilt sandwich in a grid formation (see page 126), with lines of stitches every 3–5in (7.5–12.75cm). You do not need to knot the thread for thread basting; you can leave the loose tails on top of the quilt top.

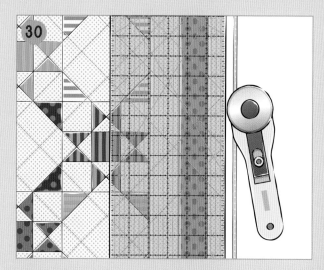

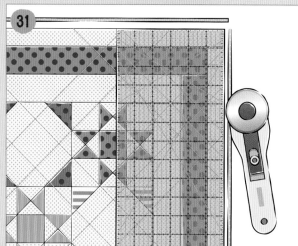

SQUARING UP & STAY-STITCHING

Once you have finished quilting (either by hand or machine) you will need to trim away the excess batting/wadding and backing fabric to the same size as the quilt top, and square up all three layers. You will also need to stay-stitch around the edge of the quilt – 'stay-stitching' is sewing generous-sized stitches close to the edge of the quilt, to hold the layers of the quilt sandwich together before adding the binding.

To square up, use either a large ruler and rotary cutter on a mat, or simply lay the quilt on a table or the floor and use fabric scissors. If you are not using a rotary cutter, we recommend drawing the cutting lines first with the help of a ruler, then trimming along these lines with your scissors.

30 To trim the sides and top and bottom edges of the quilt, lay the ruler along one edge of the quilt top and trim away the excess. It may be necessary to trim away a slight bit of the quilt top at certain points to make it square.

31 To trim the corners of the quilt, place the ruler at the corners to make a right angle and continue trimming all around the quilt.

32 To stay-stitch, after trimming sew all around the edge of the quilt with a ⅛in (3mm) seam allowance, using a stitch length of 5.0.

Behind the Snowball block name

The Snowball block is another classic American quilt block from the 19th century, and is found in many Amish quilts from that period. Its name comes from the shape of the large, corner-less square in the centre of the block. It's a very versatile block, as changing the colour of the centre patch gives the block a completely different effect.

BINDING

Binding your quilt is the final process and is a bit like adding a picture frame to your quilt. The first part is done by machine and then it is hand stitched to the back of the quilt.

33 Position two of the 2¼in (5.75cm) binding strips at a right angle, with a slight overhang and RS together. Pin the layers together. Draw a diagonal line, as shown in the illustration, then stitch along the drawn line.

34 Trim away the overhang, ¼in (5mm) away from the line you've just stitched.

35 Press the seam allowances open (**35a**), then trim the corners of the seam allowance so they're flush with the long edges of the binding (**35b**).

36 Continue joining binding strips in the same way, making sure you always add the new strip in the same direction to prevent twisting. Once you've joined all strips together, press the binding in half, WS together, along its length.

37 Lay the binding around the edges of the quilt top to make sure that no seams will meet with the corners of the quilt, as this will create too much bulk. Start along one of the edges (it doesn't matter which one), not too near to a corner.

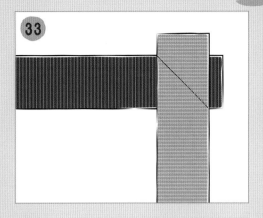

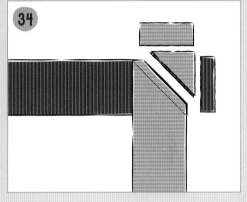

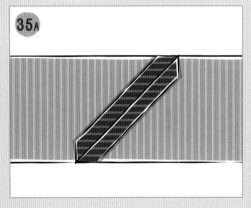

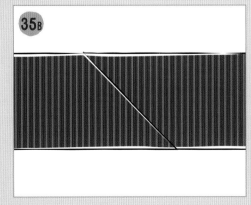

38 Once you are happy with the placement, align the raw edges of the quilt and the binding. You will be starting your stitching approx. 6in (15.25cm) away from the end of the binding, indicated by the pin in the illustration. Using a stitch length of 3.0, sew ¼in (5mm) away from the raw edges of the binding and quilt top, making sure to backstitch at the beginning (see page 124).

39 Continue sewing until you are ¼in (5mm) away from the first corner. Stop sewing, backstitch then cut the threads. Remove the quilt from under the presser foot.

40 Turn the binding up and away from the quilt top at a right angle, as shown in the illustration.

41 Then lay the binding down along the next edge of the quilt, as shown in the illustration. This will make a mitred corner. Along this next edge, start sewing ¼in (5mm) away from the first corner, making sure to backstitch at the beginning to make the stitching at the corner secure.

42 Continue around the quilt in the same way, making a mitre at each corner. Stop stitching when you are approx. 10in (25.5cm) from where you started stitching the binding.

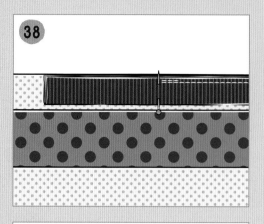

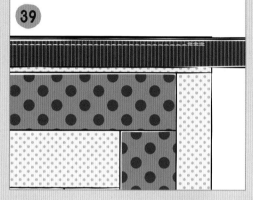

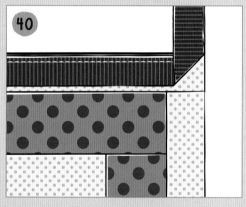

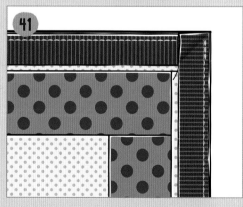

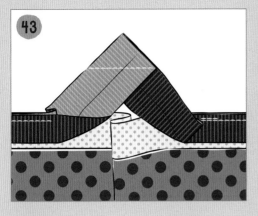

43 Overlap the two unjoined ends of the binding then trim away the excess so that they overlap by 2¼in (5.75cm). Unfold the binding ends then pin them RS together. Draw a 45-degree diagonal line across the ends, as shown in the illustration. Sew along the drawn line.

44 Open up the binding to make sure it is going to fit the quilt top exactly before trimming away the excess fabric, ¼in (5mm) away from the stitched line. Press the seam allowance open.

45 Refold the binding WS together again, then lay it flat against the quilt. Finish sewing the binding to the quilt top, joining the two ends of the stitching around the quilt and securing the final section of the binding.

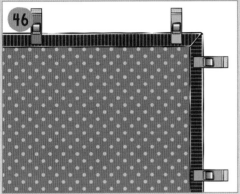

46 Fold the binding over to the back of the quilt, sandwiching the edges of the quilt inside and creating a neat mitre at each corner. Clip in place.

47 Sew the edge of the binding to the back of the quilt by hand using slip stitch (see page 126). Make sure to match the thread to the binding fabric rather than the quilt backing.

48 Sew on a label to show everyone you made a quilt! See pages 142–144 for inspiration.

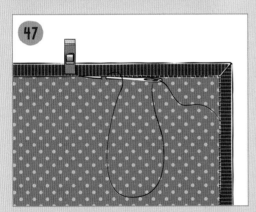

TIPS & TECHNIQUES

In this chapter of the book, we'll cover the key things about sewing that are good to know before you get stuck in. Note that specific techniques used in the projects are covered in their individual pattern instructions.

While the projects in this book are suitable for experienced sewists as well as beginners, we've tried to make sure this section is a helping hand if you're completely new to stitching: every woman, regardless of ability, should enjoy the incredibly creative and rewarding experience of sewing, in all its forms!

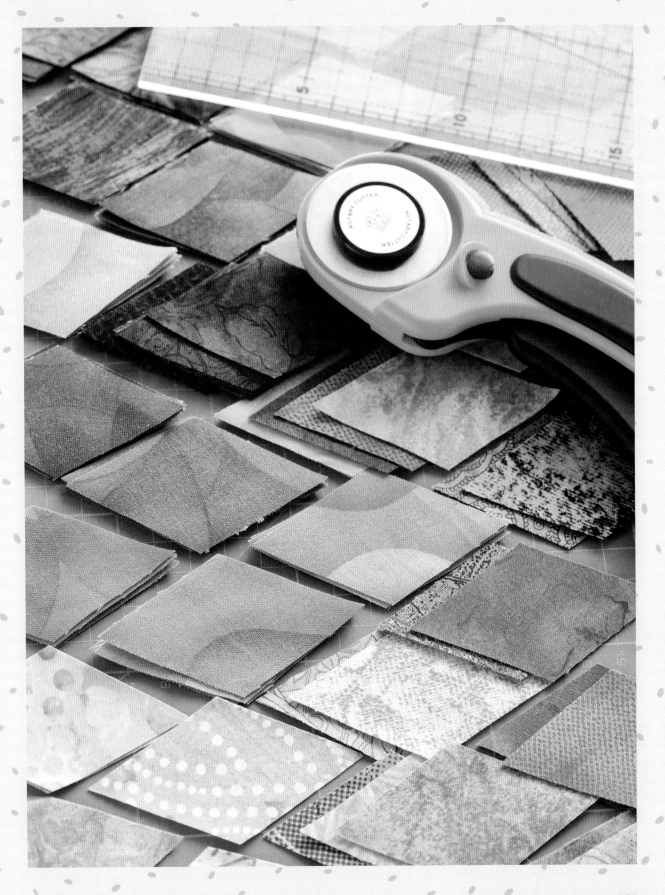

FABRIC ANATOMY

Before cutting or sewing, it's useful to understand how fabric is made and sold, so you can confidently buy your fabrics online or in person, and accurately cut out your pattern pieces too.

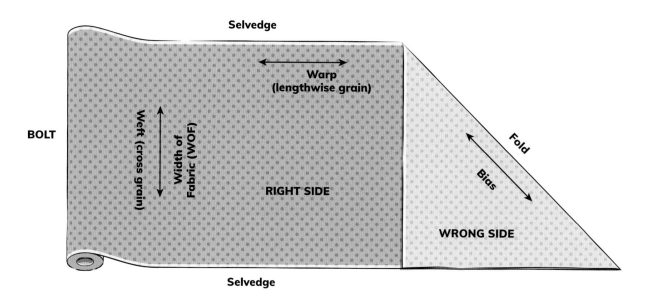

BOLT

Most manufacturers create their fabrics as long strips of cloth, which they then store and distribute neatly by wrapping them around a cardboard tube. These wrapped cloths are called **bolts**. If you go to a fabric store, you'll often see them arranged on shelves for customers to browse through in-person; you'll then request a member of staff to cut you a length from a bolt, to use for your project. Usually, you will need to purchase a minimum of a ¼yd (0.25m).

The length and width of a bolt will vary depending on the manufacturer. The average bolt is usually around 100yd (94.5m) long, and the typical widths are 44in (112cm), 54in (137.5cm) and 60in (152.5cm).

Some patterns, especially those for quilting and patchwork, will ask you to cut a piece of fabric that's a certain measurement by 'width of fabric' (**WOF**). This means the piece should be as long as the detailed measurement then as wide as the fabric bolt (the pattern will state the width of the bolt the pattern designer used).

SELVEDGES

To prevent the longer edges of the bolt from fraying and unravelling, the manufacturer will finish them in a certain way that effectively 'locks' the threads of the fabric. These finished edges are called **selvedges** (or **selvages**), and typically these are trimmed off before you start cutting out your pattern pieces.

Depending on the size of the selvedges and your seam allowance, sometimes you can make the most of your fabric by not trimming off the selvedges but cunningly sewing your fabrics so that their selvedges are hidden in the seam allowance.

Selvedges are a good way to identify the **grain** of your fabric, since they always run parallel to the **warp** threads.

FABRIC GRAIN

WARP & WEFT

Woven fabrics (i.e. fabrics that are made on a loom, like cotton) are made by weaving horizontal threads (**weft** threads) over and under vertical threads (**warp** threads), creating a **fabric grain**. The grain along the length of the fabric (i.e. parallel to the warp threads) is often known as the lengthwise grain, and the horizontal grain (parallel to the weft threads) is known as the cross grain.

If you are using patterns or templates, and you need to lay these on your fabric and cut around them, often you'll find a **grain line arrow** printed on each template piece – this arrow indicates that you need to position your template so that the arrow runs parallel to the lengthwise grain. By matching the lengthwise grain and arrow, you'll minimize fabric distortion and cut out your fabric pieces accurately. We'd only recommend cutting your fabric with the arrow running parallel to the cross grain if you're trying to save fabric.

BIAS

If you fold the fabric at a diagonal angle, then tug the fabric at both corners of the diagonal, you'll notice a little bit of stretchiness. This diagonal in the fabric is known as the **bias**. Some more complex dressmaking patterns will ask you to cut out pattern pieces on the bias, as the stretchiness creates a lovely drape in the fabric. Cutting and sewing on the bias can be tricky, however: the stretchiness means it's easy to distort or shift the fabric unintentionally, leading to inaccurately cut or seamed projects.

Some of the patchwork projects in this book will involve cutting or sewing on the bias. In these instances, we recommend using lots of pins or clips if you're joining a diagonal edge to another piece, sewing slowly, and not pulling or applying too much pressure to the fabric with your hands as you work with it.

RIGHT & WRONG SIDES

With a few exceptions (particularly 'solid' cotton fabrics that are plain on both sides), most fabrics will have a 'right side' and a 'wrong side'.

The best way to determine which side is which is by looking at how the fabric has been printed: typically manufacturers print on only one side of the fabric – this prettier side of the fabric is the **right side**. The back of the fabric, or the **wrong side**, rarely has the design printed on it.

Occasionally some of the colour printed on the front/right side of the fabric will bleed through to the back/wrong side, but the back will be much paler than the colour on the front.

ESSENTIAL MACHINE STITCHES

You'll need only a small selection of stitches to successfully make all the projects in this book, and achieve a professional finish too.

Note that you may need to adjust the stitch length (and stitch width if you're doing overcast stitch) as the ideal stitch length and width can vary from fabric to fabric. We recommend testing your stitch length on a folded scrap of your chosen fabric to start with, before stitching your actual project.

STANDARD STRAIGHT STITCH

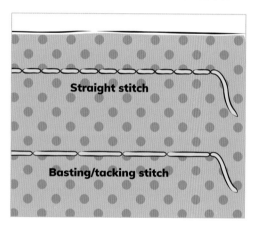

Straight stitch

Basting/tacking stitch

Every basic seam (see page 127) is stitched with a standard straight stitch. Selecting this stitch creates little running stitches with the top thread on top of your fabric that are then secured underneath with loops from the bobbin thread. By increasing the length of the stitch, you can create basting/tacking stitches.

BACKSTITCH

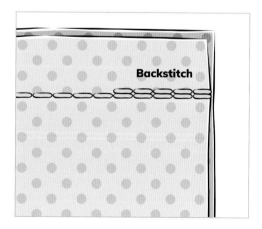

Backstitch

Unless stated otherwise, at the beginning and end of every seam you should sew backwards – known as backstitch, back-tacking or reverse stitching – as this secures both ends of the seam and stops the stitches coming undone. To stitch backwards, you will need to hold down or press a special button on your machine.

Some sewing machines have a built-in 'lock stitch' that works similarly to backstitch: it sews a single stitch backwards and forwards, then stops the machine. This creates a slightly neater, less bulky finish.

OVERCAST STITCH

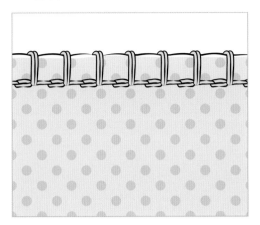

For fabrics that are likely to fray, and/or need extra security at the seams, we recommend sewing the seam allowances with overcast stitch. This will not only 'lock' the edges of the fabric, but give them a professional finish too. You will need to trim the edges of your seam allowances before stitching, to remove overhanging threads and even out the fabric if it's shifted after seaming.

If you don't have overcast stitch on your sewing machine, you can use zigzag stitch as an alternative. If you own a serger/overlocker, this can be used instead.

TOP–STITCHING

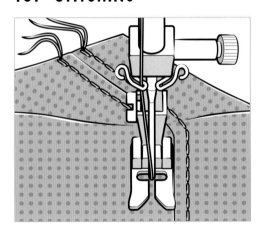

This is a stitch that serves both a decorative and practical purpose. Top-stitching is a line of stitching sewn from the right side of the fabric, usually within ¼in (5mm) of a seam, either on one or both sides. The stitching helps flatten the section around the seam, and if sewn with a contrasting thread colour adds a little embellishment to the seam too.

EDGE–STITCHING

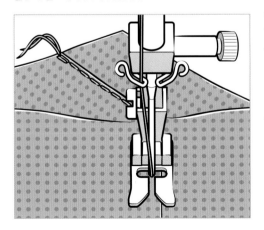

This is very similar to top-stitching, but with a few differences. The stitch line is sewn much closer to the seam – ⅛in (3mm) away – and typically a matching thread is used to hide the stitches as much as possible. This is because it serves more of a functional purpose than top-stitching: either it is used to flatten a seam, giving it a crisp edge; or, if the stitch length is increased and then sewn within the seam allowance, it temporarily secures layers of fabric in place without adding bulk if more additions are to be sewn in later.

ESSENTIAL HAND STITCHES

It is very likely you'll have come across all of these at some point in your life – whether it was at school, or if you've been mending clothes!

These core hand stitches have been used for a selection of the projects in this book, but are valuable to know for any future sewing adventures too.

RUNNING STITCH

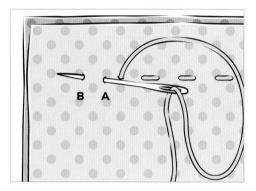

The first stitch many of us will have learned! Bring the needle up then go down at A and up again at B, keeping the stitches and the gaps between them even. Once you're confident, you can 'wiggle' the needle through the fabric a couple of times to work two to three running stitches at once.

Running stitch, if sewn with very small stitches, can be used like a straight stitch on a sewing machine: for sewing seams by hand. It's also used for basting/tacking (i.e. making temporary stitches to hold fabric together, that you'll then unpick later), and to gather fabric by hand too.

LADDER STITCH

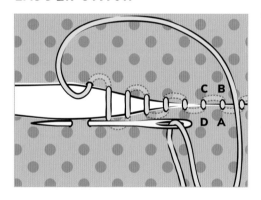

This stitch is perfect for closing openings invisibly. The right side of the fabric should be facing you, and the seam allowances of the opening should be folded inwards, to the wrong side.

Bring the needle up through one fold of the opening at A, then down directly across to the opposite side at B. A little way along, bring the needle up at C, then take it down on the opposite side at D. Repeat as necessary, keeping the stitches quite small. Every few stitches, pull the thread to pull the opening closed; the threads should 'disappear' when you do this.

SLIP STITCH

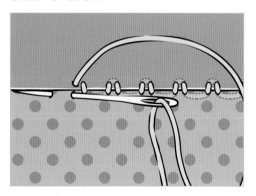

This is often used to sew a folded edge to a single layer of fabric for hemming or to finish binding, as the stitches are near invisible and very secure.

With the wrong side of the quilt or garment facing you, bury the knot inside the fold or between layers of fabric, then bring the needle and thread out through the folded edge. With the needle parallel to the folded edge, take a small stitch through the single layer of fabric directly opposite where you came out. Take a slightly longer stitch back through the fold, parallel to your previous stitch and a little way along. Repeat as necessary.

SEWING A BASIC SEAM

A seam is a secured sewn edge that's made by stitching two pieces of fabric together.

Typically, the fabrics are aligned at an edge, with the right sides of the fabric facing each other. Pin, clip or baste/tack the fabrics together at this stage, so they don't move when you sew them later on.

1 Place the fabrics in the sewing machine, at one end and with the edge to be stitched under the presser foot. Position the fabric so the needle is at the distance of the desired seam allowance (usually ¼in/5mm or ⅝in/1.5cm).

2 Start by backstitching (see page 124), then sew from one end to the other (**A**). Try to make the stitch line as straight as possible, as this will impact the size of the seam allowance and the main area of fabric, and affect how well other pieces are attached later. Before cutting the threads, backstitch at the end of your seam.

3 Open out the joined fabrics, then press the seam from the right side (see page 129). Turn over the joined fabrics so the wrong side is facing you. Depending on the project, you will need to press your seam either open (as seen in **B**) or to one side. Once the allowance is pressed, press the whole seam from the wrong side of the fabric once more.

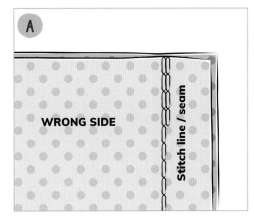

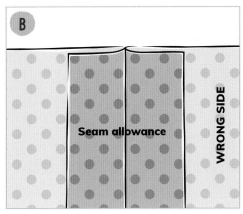

PIVOTING AT CORNERS

When sewing right-angled corners we recommend pivoting the fabric to ensure you create a sharp turn in your stitching.

Stitch up to the corner until you are the seam allowance distance away then stop, leaving the needle in the fabric. Lift the presser foot then rotate the fabric with your hands until your presser foot is lined up with the next edge. Drop the presser foot again then stitch the next edge as before.

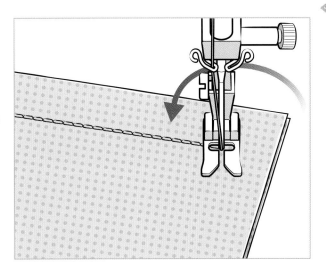

CLIPPING & NOTCHING

After sewing certain seams, you may need to clip away or notch the seam allowances to reduce bulk or help the fabric bend neatly with no fabric distortion.

Clipping away fabric at a 45-degree angle in the corners (**A**) will create sharp corners when turning the joined fabric right side out. Curved seams need help to lie flat – clip into concave curves (**B**) or notch convex curves (**C**).

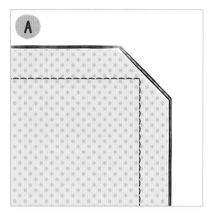

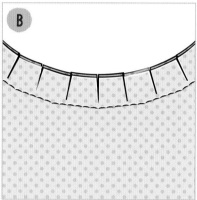

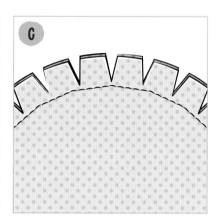

HEMS

If you are working with a single piece of fabric, and aren't sewing two pieces of fabric together, you'll almost always need to make a hem to create a neat edge, and to stop the fabric from fraying.

The two most basic hems are a single hem and a double hem. With a single hem, you turn under the fabric once (folding the fabric wrong sides together); with a double hem, you turn under the fabric twice, which sandwiches the raw edges inside a fold.

You can then either secure the hem by hand-stitching with slip stitch (see page 126), or by top-stitching on the right side of the fabric (see page 125).

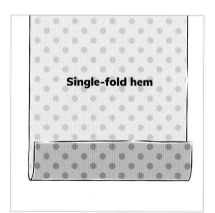

Single-fold hem

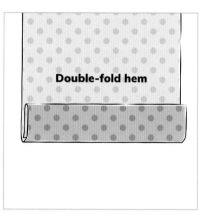

Double-fold hem

PRESSING

It's very important to press after sewing a seam, to ensure the fabric is as flat as possible for the next stage and to make the finished result look professional.

Pressing is different from ironing. With ironing, you move the iron around on the fabric; with pressing, the iron is literally pressed against the fabric with no movement, held there for a few seconds, then the action is repeated at another point on the fabric (**A**).

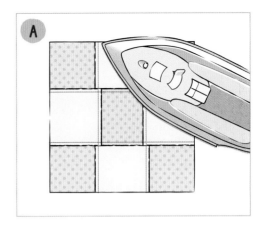

As some fabrics will be sensitive to the heat, or will melt if they directly touch an iron, we recommend investing in a pressing cloth (**B**). To use a pressing cloth, simply place it over the fabric to be pressed then press as normal. If you need steam, dampen the cloth before placing it on top of your fabric. Always use a pressing cloth to apply fusible interfacing to your fabric, as it will help the interfacing adhere to the fabric more quickly and evenly.

When sewing patchwork pieces together, it's important every seam is pressed before it is crossed by another.

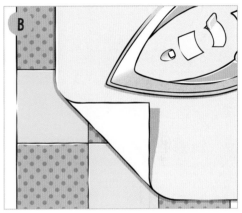

To reduce bulk where two vertical seams meet (for example, one seam is sitting on top of another seam, with both running in the same direction), press one seam allowance to one side and the other seam allowance in the other direction. This is known as 'nesting'.

In **C**, the seam allowances in the top and bottom rows are pressed away from the centre squares, while the seam allowances in the centre row are pressed towards the centre square. When the rows are joined, the seam allowances of the rows are nested and top and bottom seam allowances are pressed in opposite directions, away from the centre row.

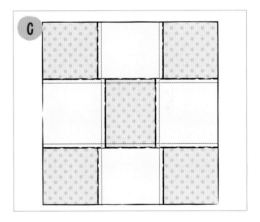

PATCHWORK & QUILTING

Some sewists are a little intimidated by patchwork and quilting, but you needn't be. Start off small (for example the Log Cabin Placemats on page 64), and you'll discover how wonderful this type of sewing can be.

Patchwork and quilting started off as a way to turn scraps of fabric into beautiful practical items. Although both have transformed into more complex crafts, the purpose behind them and the simple techniques involved in making them are still at their core, centuries later.

There are one or two specialized techniques, but once you've covered these, you'll be confidently stitching a quilt in no time!

PRE-CUTS

Based on the way a fabric bolt is cut, certain 'cuts' have emerged that are now universally known in the quilt world. These allow you to make the most out of a certain length of fabric, and the sizes offer a great deal of versatility.

With quilting and patchwork being as popular as it is, pre-cut fabrics can be purchased more and more easily at hobby stores. While there are many more pre-cuts available than what is shown below, these are the main ones used in this book.

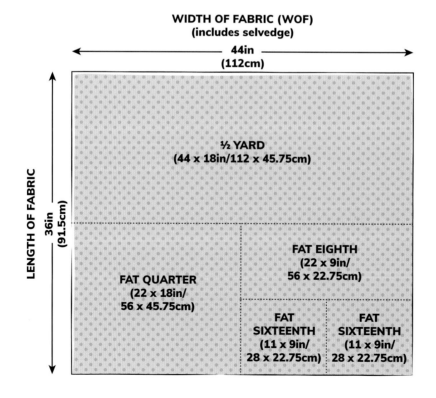

WIDTH OF FABRIC (WOF)
(includes selvedge)

44in
(112cm)

LENGTH OF FABRIC

36in
(91.5cm)

½ YARD
(44 x 18in/112 x 45.75cm)

FAT EIGHTH
(22 x 9in/
56 x 22.75cm)

FAT QUARTER
(22 x 18in/
56 x 45.75cm)

FAT SIXTEENTH
(11 x 9in/
28 x 22.75cm)

FAT SIXTEENTH
(11 x 9in/
28 x 22.75cm)

ROTARY CUTTING

When it comes to cutting your fabric for patchwork, we recommend using a rotary cutter, cutting mat and ruler. This makes the process much quicker and more accurate. On page 24 we've provided some information on what equipment to invest in for rotary cutting.

Before cutting out any fabrics, always double-check what fabrics to cut into, the measurements and cutting amounts. There's nothing worse than cutting out lots of pieces, and realizing you've cut out too many pieces, the fabrics are the wrong size, you've used the wrong fabric – or all three!

1 To start, you'll need your chosen rotary cutter, cutting mat and quilting ruler.

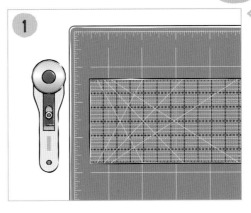

2 If you need to straighten up your fabric edges: place the fabric to be cut on the cutting mat, lining up the selvedge edge with a horizontal line on the cutting mat. Lay the ruler on top of the fabric, slightly in from the edge of the fabric and aligning the edge of the ruler with a vertical line on the mat. Trim the edge from bottom to top – cutting away from yourself – in one fluid motion and pressing gently but firmly on the cutter.

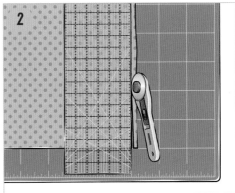

3 To cut strips: align the fabric with a vertical line on the mat, then place the ruler parallel to the edge of the fabric to be cut, positioning it away from the fabric edge at the desired width. Cut from bottom to top. For longer cuts, keep a consistent pressure on the cutter and ruler but gradually move your hand on the ruler farther away from you, as you work upwards.

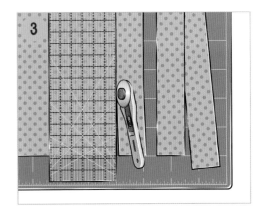

4 To cut multiple squares: cut the strip as in Step 3. Lay the strip horizontally over the cutting mat, lining up the end with a vertical line on the mat. Place the ruler over the strip, until you have your desired measurement. Cut from bottom to top. Repeat along the whole strip.

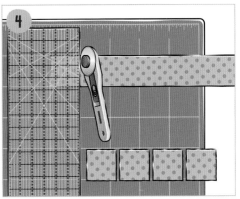

QUILTING

Quilting is the stitching used to join together the three layers of the quilt sandwich while adding a decorative element too. It can be done either by hand or machine and we have used both methods in this book.

MARKING

Before any quilting is done, we recommend marking out your quilt pattern. This will not only give you nice guides to follow, but will help you get an overview of the whole design too.

On page 24 of this book, we noted several marking tools you could use for the marking process:

- water-soluble fabric marker pen (**A**),
- fabric pencil or chalk pencil (**B**),
- hera marker (**C**).

Always test your preferred marking tool on a scrap of fabric first.

Often it is possible to use the seams of your quilt blocks as a guide for your stitching, depending how far apart you would like the quilting lines to be. However, if the quilt has borders you will need to mark at least the lines extending into the borders to know where to start and end your quilting.

If you have a walking (dual-/even-feed) foot, it may well come with a quilting guide bar that can be adjusted to different widths; this is very helpful when it comes to stitching parallel lines that are always the same distance from each other (**D**).

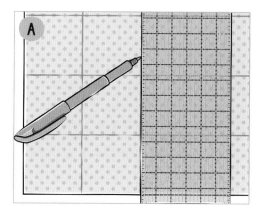

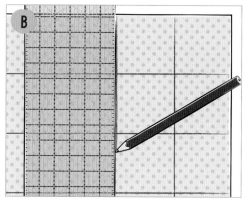

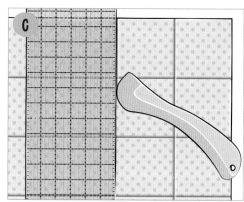

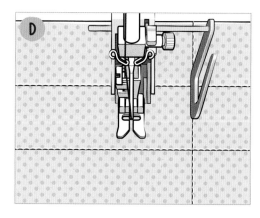

WHAT THREAD TO USE FOR QUILTING?

Different weights of quilting thread will give different finished effects. For the Log Cabin Placemats (see page 64), we suggest using a heavy-weight thread to give the quilting more of a 'rustic' look, and to add texture. For the Keep Cool Quilt (see page 106), you can use a finer weight thread if you wish.

A 50wt cotton thread will 'melt' into the project, giving a delicate line; 40wt cotton thread will add a bit more definition to the quilting, and 28wt will create bold stitching. All of these can be stitched by hand or machine. A 12wt or perle cotton can be used for quilting too, but is best used for hand quilting.

WHAT NEEDLES TO USE FOR QUILTING?

- 50wt or 40wt thread with John James Sharps or quilting needles in size 10
- 12wt thread with John James Embroidery needles in size 3 or 5.

For machine quilting, we like to use:

- 50wt or 40wt thread with an 80/12 needle
- 28wt thread with a 90/14 needle.

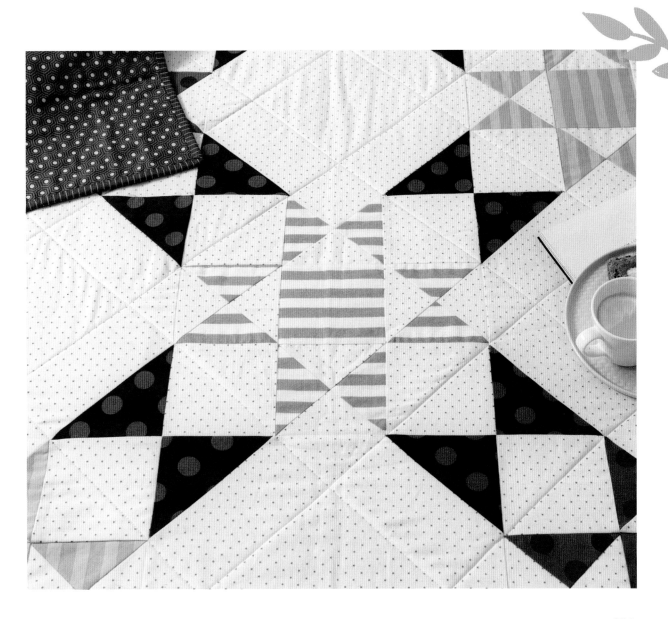

HAND QUILTING

Use running stitch for all hand quilting (see page 126). It's important to note that, as both sides of the quilt will be visible, all the thread ends where you start and finish need to be hidden between the layers of the quilt sandwich.

It is worth making up a small sample quilt sandwich approximately 12in (30.5cm) square to practise your quilting, before committing to a full-size quilt. Some quilters like to use a quilters' hoop when hand quilting; however, this is optional.

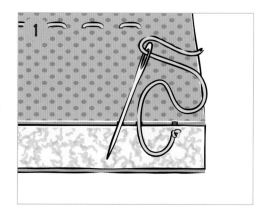

1 Always start quilting from the centre of your quilt working outwards. Thread an approx. 14–16in (35.5–40.75cm) length of thread on your needle and make a knot in the end. About ⅜in (1cm) away from where you'd like your quilting to start, insert the needle through the quilt top into the batting/wadding – do not take it through to the backing. Bring the needle up where you intend to start stitching. Pull the thread gently until the knot on top of the quilt top 'pops' under it.

2 Make your first running stitch, taking the needle through all three layers of your quilt sandwich.

3 Continue with running stitch for the rest of your quilt design, going through all three layers of the quilt sandwich, and trying to make the stitches as even in length as possible on both the front and back. The lines of quilting should go all the way to the edge of the quilt top. If using a lighter weight thread, your stitches will normally be smaller than if using a heavy-weight thread. However, the stitch length is personal and will depend on the look you desire.

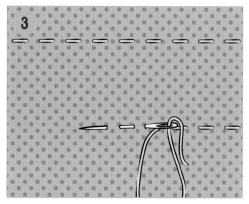

Depending on your confidence with stitching and the thickness of your batting/wadding, you may find you can make two or more stitches at a time (see the illustration).

4 Either when your thread runs out or as you come to the end of a row of stitches, finish off by making a knot on the remainder of your thread. Make a stitch by inserting the needle back into the quilt top and batting/wadding and coming out about 1in (2.5cm) away, pulling the knot underneath the quilt top as in Step 1. Snip the thread close to the quilt top. If needed, bury the end by easing it beneath the surface with the tip of your needle.

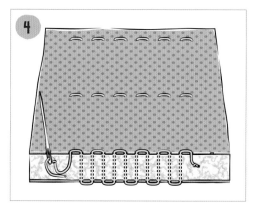

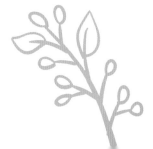

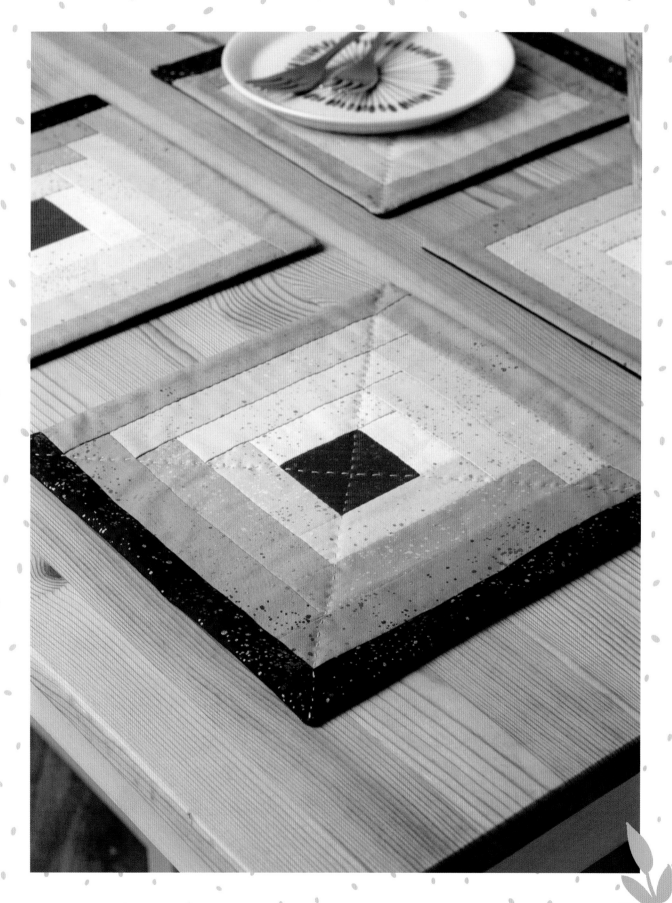

MACHINE QUILTING

It is possible to quilt a large quilt (such as the Keep Cool Quilt on page 106) on a standard domestic sewing machine. Quilting on a machine can be more time efficient than hand quilting, and the density of stitching offers a different look.

For our Keep Cool Quilt, we have suggested straight-line quilting in an edge-to-edge style, which means that there is no stopping and starting within the quilt top.

There are a couple of optional tools that can make the process easier:

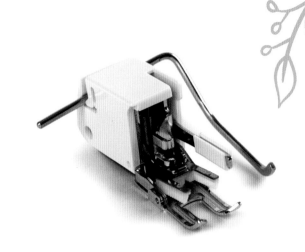

- **Walking foot (dual-/even-feed):** This can be purchased for most sewing machines. This foot has its own set of feed dogs that work with the feed dogs on the machine, pulling multiple layers of fabric through evenly – perfect for quilts. It also prevents slipping, and helps create even quilt stitches too.

- **Extension table:** This may come as an accessory with your machine. It extends the working surface (hence the name), and helps keep the quilt supported while it's being stitched.

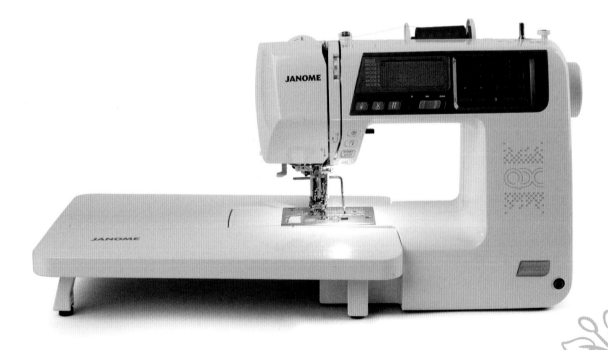

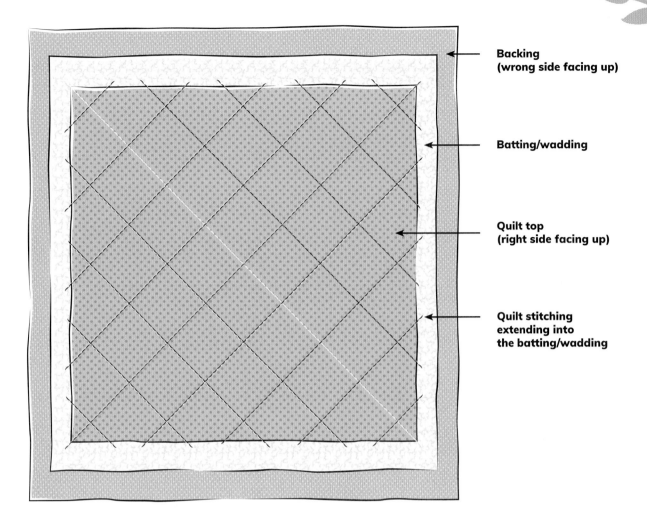

**Backing
(wrong side facing up)**

Batting/wadding

**Quilt top
(right side facing up)**

**Quilt stitching
extending into
the batting/wadding**

Note: Use a stitch length of 3.0 if using a 40wt or 50wt thread. You might want to use a longer stitch length of 3.5 if you are using a heavier thread.

1 Start quilting by stitching across one of the central diagonals of the quilt sandwich (see the yellow and pink stitch lines) or one of the straight lines that run through the centre of the quilt (horizontal or vertical), from one corner (or side) to the other. Begin your stitching beyond the edge of the quilt top, in the batting/wadding approx. ½in (1.25cm) away from the quilt top, then end your stitch line in the batting/wadding at the opposite corner (or side). Backstitch at the start and end of the stitch line, at the edge of the quilt top so it sits within the ¼in (5mm) seam allowance; this central stitching will help prevent any puckering or bunching of the fabric, and keep the quilt flat.

2 To stitch your next line, lift the machine foot and needle and re-position the quilt sandwich at your desired distance from the previous stitch line. Backstitch, then stitch your line, quilting across the quilt top into the batting/wadding at the opposite corner (or side). Backstitch to finish off.

3 Repeat Step 2 until you've added stitch lines to the whole quilt. From the centre stitch line, we like to fill in one corner (or side) of the quilt then fill in the other corner (or side); we find this makes rotating the quilt less cumbersome.

DRESSMAKING

We've included two garments in this book – the Cool-down Cover-up (see page 94) and Maker's Apron (see page 86) – that are gorgeous, practical and achievable to make, ideal if you are fresh to dressmaking. If you haven't made any clothes before, here is some useful information to get you started.

SIZING & MEASURING

The size chart for both the Keep Cool Cover-up and Maker's Apron is provided below. Measure your body then refer to the chart below to decide which size to sew.

If you've not measured yourself before, you'll need to wear light clothing or just your underwear, and have a tape measure. If you need help getting an accurate measurement, you can ask a 'measuring buddy' to assist you.

We've included the key measurements in the diagram opposite, plus some extras that are important to know if you decide to dive deeper into the world of dressmaking!

UK size	US size	Size marked on template sheets	Bust measurement (circum.)	Hip measurement (circum.)
8–10	4–6	S–M	37⅜in (95cm)	39⅜in (100cm)
12–14	8–10	L–XL	39⅜in (100cm)	42½in (108cm)
16–18	12–14	XXL	42½in (108cm)	46in (117cm)
20–22	16–18	3XL	46in (117cm)	49⅝in (126cm)
24	20	4XL	49⅝in (126cm)	53⅛in (135cm)
26	22	5XL	53⅛in (135cm)	56¾in (144cm)
28	24	6XL	56¾in (144cm)	60⅝in (154cm)

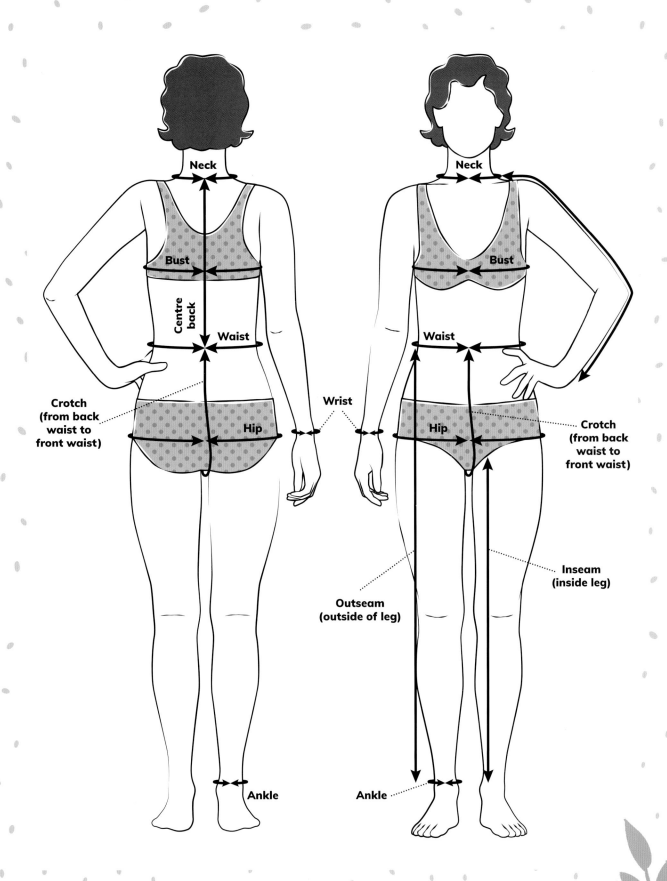

Neck

Bust

Centre back

Waist

Crotch (from back waist to front waist)

Hip

Wrist

Ankle

Neck

Bust

Waist

Crotch (from back waist to front waist)

Hip

Inseam (inside leg)

Outseam (outside of leg)

Ankle

UNDERSTANDING PATTERNS

Dressmaking patterns can have their own language; below are the things you'll need to know for most patterns, and for those included in this book.

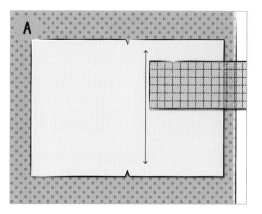

- **Grain line:** This is the direction of the fabric weave. On the dressmaking patterns, a grain line is indicated by a long arrow (**A**); this needs to run parallel to the selvedge of the fabric, to ensure that the finished garment will drape properly.

- **Notches:** These can indicate many things in a pattern, but more often than not they act as 'balance points' – marks that help you position and sew the right pieces together – and will often appear on long or curved seams for this reason.

  Notches can also indicate features on garments like pleats, or the key points on a pattern such as the centre back.

  Notches appear as small lines or triangles on commercial patterns. You cut your notches as you're cutting out your fabric pieces. There are four ways you can cut your notches: you can either 'mirror' the triangle shape by cutting an extra triangle beyond the seam allowance (**B**, top); cut a triangle into the seam allowance (**B**, middle); make a slit in the seam allowance (**B**, bottom); or simply mark with an erasable pen.

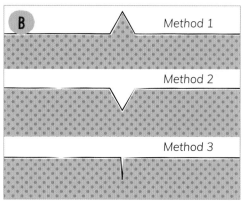

Method 1

Method 2

Method 3

- **Cutting on the fold:** To ensure you have a neat and symmetrical cut, some patterns will ask you to cut pieces 'on the fold' – this means folding your fabric in half, right sides together, then aligning the indicated edge of the pattern with the fold.

- **Pattern layout:** Some patterns will provide you with information on how to position the pattern pieces on your chosen fabric, maximizing your cut of fabric as much as possible – the example seen in **C** features the pattern pieces for the Maker's Apron. Most pattern layouts suit a standard 44in (112cm) wide bolt of fabric; however, occasionally it will give guidance on laying out your patterns on alternative fabric widths, so choose the one that matches the fabric you are using. If your pattern doesn't come with layout information, arrange all your pattern pieces on your fabric before cutting anything out, to ensure you make the most out of your fabric.

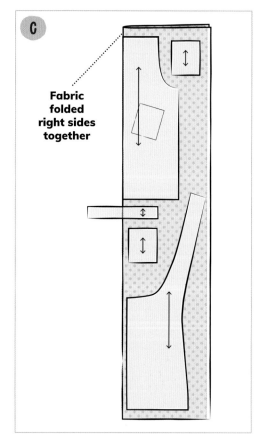

Fabric folded right sides together

"There is nothing more rare, nor more beautiful, than a woman being unapologetically herself."

DR. STEVE MARABOLI

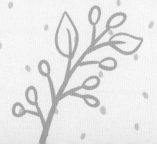

ADDING LABELS

Here is our simple guide to labelling your finished projects. This doesn't have to be a time-consuming or expensive addition. It is your opportunity to celebrate reaching the finish line, which we know is not always easy when life gets in the way!

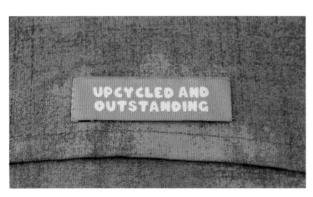

'Upcycled and Outstanding'

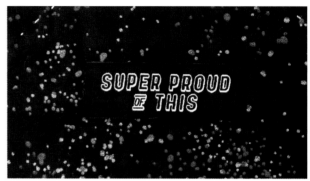

'Super Proud of This'

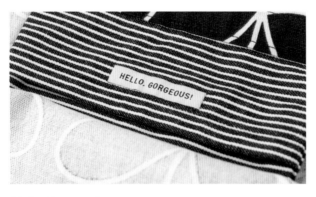

'Hello, Gorgeous!'

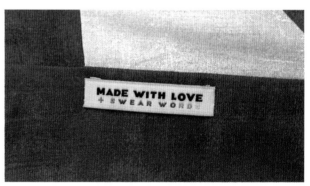

'Made with Love + Swear Words'

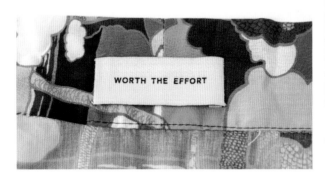

'Worth the Effort'

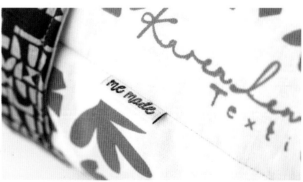

'Me Made'

SMALL PROJECTS & GARMENTS

The two main options here are:

- To purchase bespoke woven labels which come in many different styles and identify you as the maker. They can be especially poignant if you are gifting one of your *Menopause Makes* projects.

- To purchase woven labels with a design or slogan that makes you smile.

The labels opposite, by Kylie and The Machine, are some of our favourites.

Depending on the style of label you choose, it will be attached either during construction (for example, between two layers of fabric that will be stitched together so it's trapped in the seam – see **A–C** below) or upon completion of the project. If using small 'end fold' labels (like the ones you see at the neckline of a garment) it is easier to secure with hand stitching.

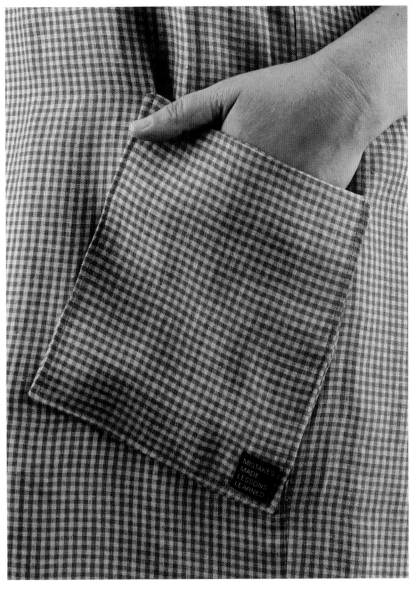

'Mistakes Made Lessons Learned'

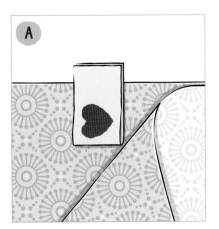

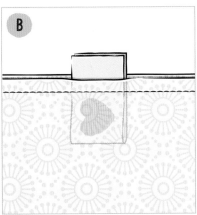

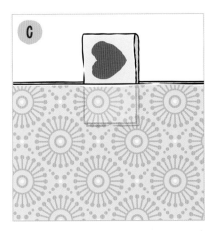

QUILT LABELS

As the saying goes 'Anonymous was a woman'!

However, we do not want you, our menopause makers, and your beautiful work to go unnoticed in the future, especially as quilts are big investments of time and effort and will become family heirlooms.

The simplest way to attach a label to your quilt is to write on a piece of fabric and sew it onto your quilt (a piece measuring approximately 5 x 4in/12.75 x 10cm is a good size).

Start with a scrap of your chosen fabric, then test a permanent fabric pen on it to make sure the ink doesn't bleed. Once you're satisfied with the result, write out your label's message, leaving a border of at least 1in (2.5cm) all around it.

What to include:

- Date it was made (don't worry if it stretches over several years!).

- The maker's name – you!

- Who it was made for (even if it is a gift to yourself).

- Where it was made.

- Any other message or information you would like to include.

Using your own handwriting in this way adds a personal touch to your quilt.

If your stitching skills are up to it, you could hand embroider over your handwritten words, or use the embroidery feature on your machine if you have one – this is what we used in the label for our Keep Cool Quilt (see page 106), seen in the example below.

Add more embellishment to your label by drawing, using hand or machine embroidery, or sewing on decorative patches – we added a tiny woven label in the example below.

Once you are happy with the label, turn under the edges by ½in (1.25cm) all the way around and sew it to to the back of your quilt with slip stitch. Ensure your stitches are not visible on the quilt top. A label is traditionally placed in one of the bottom corners.

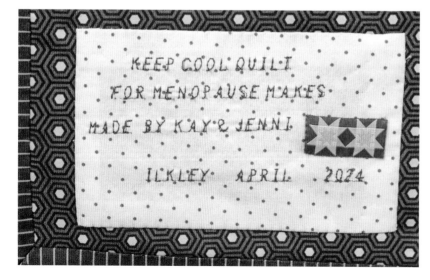

*'Keep Cool Quilt
for Menopause Makes*

Made by Kay & Jenni

Ilkley April 2024'

"*Creativity is inventing, experimenting, growing, taking risks, breaking rules, making mistakes, and having fun.*"

MARY LOU COOK

RESOURCES

Here are some useful websites for finding sewing supplies and learning more about our Guest Designers.

SUPPLIERS

- **Aurifil**
  Thread.
  aurifil.com

- **Ernest Wright**
  Scissors.
  ernestwright.co.uk

- **Janome**
  Sewing machines.
  janome.co.uk/janome.com

- **Kylie and The Machine**
  Woven labels.
  kylieandthemachine.com

- **Liberty™**
  Fabrics and haberdashery.
  libertylondon.com

- **Olfa**
  Rotary cutters, cutting mats and rulers.
  olfa.co.uk/olfa.com

- **Vlieseline**
  Interfacings and interlinings.
  vlieseline.com

- **Warm Company**
  Quilt batting/wadding.
  warmcompany.com

GUEST DESIGNERS

- **Alice Garrett**
  See pages 104 and 105.
  alicecaroline.com

- **Karen Lewis**
  See pages 46 and 47.
  karenlewistextiles.com

- **Rashida Coleman-Hale**
  See pages 62 and 63.
  rashidacolemanhale.com
  AND
  rubystarsociety.com

- **Sally Kelly**
  See pages 38 and 39.
  sallykelly.london
  AND
  windhamfabrics.com

THANKS &
ACKNOWLEDGEMENTS

There has been a rather magical momentum during the making of this book: an infectious enthusiasm and excitement from people, knowing that together we are breaking new ground in the crafting sphere and truly want to make a difference to menopausal women everywhere.

Thank you Samantha Warrington and David Grant at Search Press for your warm reception to our pitch and for sweeping into action! You gave us an exceptional team who have brought our vision to life better than we could have hoped for. Emily Adam, thank you for your attention to detail, passion and patience. Nobody writes a more precise email than you! Marrianne (Maz) Miall, thank you for your fresh and innovative design – your dedication to make this book a joy to look at was evident from our very first call. Thank you also to Stacy Grant for the styled photography and to Mark Davison and Becky Robbins for a wonderful shoot day in the studio. We also love the illustrations throughout the book by Kuo Kang Chen; thank you so much.

It was definitely a 'pinch us' moment when we heard that Rashida Coleman-Hale had accepted the brief to design the book's cover, and she captured the vibe of community, fun and creativity so perfectly. Thank you Rashida, and our other guest designers Sally Kelly, Karen Lewis and Alice Garrett for sharing your personal insights in these pages, and for making our stitching world so much brighter.

A late but very happy addition to the book was when our Liberty™ muse Alison Lewis agreed to model some of our makes: Alison, your smile is infectious and you are a true proponent of handmade style; we are so glad that you said yes! Thank you also to Nomeda Padskociute-Lukosiuniene for your wonderful pattern-cutting and advice on the garments in the book.

Thank you to Deborah Shepherd and the team at Janome for believing in this project and producing machines we love to sew on each day. Thank you to our Aurifil family too, especially Bradley Mitchell, Alex Winton and Erin Sampson; your thread is woven into every one of our projects and your friendship has been invaluable over the past 10 years.

The 'What is the Menopause?' foreword by Hannah Davies is very insightful, and provides the perfect start to this book. A huge thank you, Hannah, for sharing your knowledge and expertise with all of us.

And finally a big thank you to our family and friends for listening and caring so much about the work that we do.

GLOSSARY

> **Basting/tacking**
Temporarily holding layers of fabric together, to stop them from moving. This can be with stitches, basting spray or pins. See page 115 for more information.

> **Block**
A patchwork square that is a design in itself, which is usually joined to other blocks to make into a quilt.

> **Bolt**
– A long strip of finished cloth rolled up around a cardboard tube.

– For domestic small-scale sewing, you will instruct a shop to cut specific lengths from a bolt (the minimum length usually being ¼yd or 0.25m.

– The width of a bolt can vary considerably. Typically, quilting fabric is 44in (112cm) wide, while many dressmaking fabrics are 45in (115cm), 54–55in (137–140cm) or 60in (152cm). We recommend strongly to check the pattern requirements before you buy your fabric.

> **Edge-stitch(ing)**
This is a line of stitching sewn close to a seam – approximately ⅛in (3mm) away – to help create a crisp edge.

> **Flying Geese**
A type of patchwork block or unit (see page 73).

> **Hourglass**
A type of patchwork block or unit (see page 110).

> **HST(s)**
Half Square Triangle(s), a type of patchwork block or unit (see pages 80 and 110).

> **Log Cabin**
A type of patchwork block or unit (see page 68).

> **Nesting seams**
Especially important in patchwork, this is aligning the seams and making sure the seam allowances fit together.

> **Ohio Star**
A type of patchwork block or unit (see page 111).

> **Piecing**
The process of sewing multiple patchwork shapes together, to make a unit or block.

> **Pivot**
Turning a corner sharply when sewing, raising the presser foot but keeping the needle in the fabric to ensure the fabric doesn't shift.

> **Press**
This is different to 'ironing' – simply place the iron on the section instructed for a few seconds, without moving the iron. This flattens the area, and removes wrinkles.

> **Quilt sandwich**
The three layers of a quilt – backing on the bottom, batting/wadding in the middle, and the quilt top on top.

> **Raw edges**
As it sounds: the raw, cut edges of the fabric. You should match or align these when stitching a seam, so there is no distortion in the fabric of the joined pieces.

> **RS**
Right side(s) of the fabric, i.e. the 'pretty' front side of the fabric.

> Seam allowance
– The area between the raw, cut fabric edge and stitching line. A seam allowance creates a stable seam, and stops the seam from coming apart.

– Usually, it is hidden inside the project or garment.

– When you sew two fabric pieces together, often you will press the seam allowance in a certain direction to prevent bulk or to make the seam allowance less obvious on the RS.

– A seam allowance can also be finished to prevent fraying; you can use zigzag or overcast stitch for this.

> Selvedge
Also spelled 'selvage', this refers to what is called the 'self-finished' edges on a bolt of fabric. When you purchase fabric from a bolt, you'll notice neat 'borders' (often with information about the fabric printed on them) that run down the length of the fabric edges. These stop the edges of the fabric bolt from unravelling and fraying.

> Shoo Fly
A type of patchwork block or unit (see page 81).

> Snowball
A type of patchwork block or unit (see page 112).

> Stay-stitching
Sewing generous-sized stitches close to the edge of the quilt, to help hold the layers of the quilt sandwich together before adding the binding.

> Stitch length
The size of your stitches when sewing. On a sewing machine, the stitch length can be adjusted to serve a particular purpose – from making longer stitches for basting/tacking to accommodating the fabric you're sewing (for example, light-weight fabrics need a shorter stitch length than a heavy-weight fabric).

> Top-stitch(ing)
This is a line of stitching sewn from the RS of the fabric, often close to a seam, either to help a seam sit better or to add embellishment, or both.

> Turn under
Fold over the edge of the fabric, usually so wrong sides are facing.

> Unfinished block size
The measurement of the block once all its units are stitched together, but the block is not yet stitched into the quilt (so, includes the seam allowance).

> Unit
Sometimes used synonymously with 'block', 'unit' usually refers to smaller patchwork elements that are eventually sewn into a block. For example, several units are sewn together to make a block.

> WOF
Width of fabric. This is term used to describe the width measurement of a bolt of fabric.

> WS
Wrong side(s) of the fabric, i.e. the plain back of the fabric.

INDEX

A

anxiety 7, 9, 39, 47, 76

B

backstitch 34, 42, 50, 56, 66, 96, 124, 127, 137
baste(ing) 24, 36, 57, 91, 92, 99, 103, 114, 115, 124, 126, 127, 148, 149
batting 20, 66, 108, 115, 116, 134, 137, 146, 148
binding 116, 117–119, 126, 149
bolt 20, 56, 66, 72, 78, 108, 122, 130, 140, 148, 149
border(s), quilt 72, 74, 78, 83, 113, 114, 132
brain fog 7, 9, 13, 70

C

clipping 52, 59, 75, 84, 91, 92, 102, 128
clumsiness 7, 86
cotton (fabric) 18, 20, 23, 106, 123
  – lawn 18, 96, 106
  – quilting 18, 38, 106
cutting mat 18, 24, 116, 113, 131
cutting shapes 73, 80, 110, 131

D

depression 7, 48
directional (fabric) 34, 43, 72, 74, 89, 96, 101, 111, 112
dry hair 7, 54
dry skin 7, 54
dual-feed foot see walking foot

E

edge-stitch(ing) 45, 53, 75, 90, 92, 99, 103, 125, 148
even-feed foot see walking foot

F

fabric clip(s) 23, 123
Fat Eighth 34, 42, 66, 130
Fat Quarter 42, 72, 78, 108, 130
Fat Sixteenth 66, 130
fleece 20, 34, 42, 43, 56, 60, 76, 78
Flying Geese (block) 22, 70, 72, 73, 148
French seam(s) 18, 89, 90, 98, 100, 102

G

garment(s) 18, 20, 24, 26, 27, 28, 38, 62, 86–93, 94–103, 138, 139, 140, 143, 149
grain 34, 114, 122, 123, 140
  – grain line arrow 34, 123, 140

H

Half Square Triangle (block) 76, 80, 85, 110, 148
hand-tying 76, 78, 85
hem(s) 51, 52, 75, 90, 92, 93, 101, 102, 103, 126, 128
hot flash(es) 7, 8, 13, 32, 94, 106
Hourglass (block) 109, 110, 11, 148

I

insomnia 32, 39, 106
interfacing 24, 42, 43, 56, 57, 60, 129

L

label(s) 51, 75, 91, 119, 143, 144
ladder stitch 36, 69, 84, 93, 126
linen (fabric) 18, 88, 93
Log Cabin (block) 62, 64–69, 130, 133, 148

M

marking 34, 52, 53, 57, 59, 60, 66, 73, 80, 85, 110, 112, 114, 117, 119, 132, 140, 144
  – tools 24, 66, 72, 78, 108, 132, 144
memory loss 7, 9, 13, 40, 70

N

needle(s) 18, 22, 23, 34, 50, 78, 96, 114, 126, 133, 134, 137
notch(es) 34, 36, 59, 96, 98, 99, 100, 101, 102, 140
notching 36, 101, 151

O

Ohio Star (block) 109, 111, 148
oilcloth 60
overcast stitch 52, 124, 125, 149

P

patchwork 17, 18, 20, 22, 24, 38, 62, 64–69, 70, 73, 74, 76–85, 106–119, 122, 123, 129, 130, 131, 148, 149

pin(s) 18, 23, 123

pivoting 52, 91, 127, 148

pocket(s) 48, 50, 51, 53, 86, 89, 91

polyester 18, 20

pre-cut(s) 20, 34, 42, 66, 72, 78, 108, 130

press(ing) 20, 24, 36, 43, 57, 66, 72, 78, 93, 101, 108, 127, 129, 148, 149

pressing cloth 24, 35, 43, 57, 93, 129

Q

quarter-inch (¼in) foot 22

quilt sandwich 148

quilt stitching 22, 23, 24, 66, 69, 108, 114, 132–137

R

right side 123, 127, 137, 140, 148

rotary cutter 18, 24, 80, 83, 110, 112, 113, 116, 117, 121, 131, 146

ruler 24, 80, 112, 116, 131, 146
– square 24, 78, 108, 110

running stitch 66, 115, 126, 134

S

safety pin(s) 24, 34, 35, 78, 84, 115

seam 34, 44, 50, 56, 58, 60, 66, 80, 83, 88, 96, 112, 124, 125, 127, 129, 148, 149
see also French seams

seam allowance(s) 29, 34, 42, 50, 52, 56, 66, 72, 78, 88, 96, 108, 122, 125, 126, 127, 128, 129, 137, 140, 149
– nesting 74, 82, 100, 112, 129, 148

seam gauge 24, 52, 88, 96

selvedge/selvage 83, 113, 122, 130, 131, 140, 149

sewing machine 17, 22, 45, 124, 125, 127, 144, 146

Shoo Fly (block) 78, 81, 82, 85, 149

shrinkage (fabric) 20, 83, 113

silk 18, 34, 36, 43, 57

size chart(s) 88, 96, 97, 138

slip stitch 119, 126,128, 144

Snowball (block) 112, 116, 149

standard foot 22, 44, 127, 148

stay-stitching 116, 149

stitch length 34, 42, 45, 50, 53, 56, 57, 58, 72, 78, 88, 96, 108, 116, 118, 124, 125, 134, 137, 149

straight stitch 124, 126, 127, 136, 137

strap(s) 34, 36, 48, 50, 52, 53, 90, 91, 92

strips, cutting 131

stress 9, 47, 64

sweat(ing/s) 7, 106

T

tack(ing) see baste(ing)

Tana Lawn™
see lawn under cotton

tape measure 14, 24, 138

template(s) 34, 42, 88, 89, 91, 96, 97, 123, 138, 152

thread(s) 17, 18, 23, 34, 42, 50, 56, 66, 69, 72, 78, 85, 88, 96, 108, 114, 115, 119, 124, 125, 133, 134, 137, 146

top-stitch(ing) 58, 91, 97, 125, 128, 149

W

wadding see batting

walking foot 22, 108, 118, 127, 132, 136, 137, 148
– guide bar 22, 122, 132

width of fabric (WOF) 56, 66, 72, 78, 88, 97, 108, 122, 130, 149

wrong side 89, 98, 122, 123, 126, 127, 128, 137, 149

Z

zip 54, 57, 58, 59, 60

zipper foot 22, 57, 58

First published in 2025

Search Press Limited
Wellwood, North Farm Road,
Tunbridge Wells, Kent TN2 3DR

Text and patterns copyright
© Jenni Smith and Kay Walsh

Photography
Page 27: from second image down –
magicbones/stock.adobe.com,
Alexandra/stock.adobe.com,
Steph Wilson on unsplash.com

Page 39: copyright © Sally Kelly

Page 47: copyright © Karen Lewis

Page 63: copyright © Rashida Coleman-Hale

Page 105: copyright © Alice Garrett

Stacy Grant: pages 1 (M), 5, 11, 27 (T), 33, 37,
41, 42, 50, 55, 56, 61, 65, 71, 75, 77, 79, 84, 87,
93, 107, 133 and 135. Copyright © Search Press Ltd.

Mark Davison: all remaining photographs.
Copyright © Search Press Ltd.

Illustrations
Cover artwork by Rashida Coleman-Hale

Interior illustrations by Kuo Kang Chen

Illustrations and design copyright
© Search Press Ltd.

ISBN: 978-1-80092-254-9
ebook ISBN: 978-1-80093-253-1
Pattern sheet pack: 978-1-80092-367-6

Suppliers
If you have difficulty in obtaining any of the materials
and equipment mentioned in this book, then please visit
the Search Press website for details of suppliers:

www.searchpress.com

Bookmarked
Extra, downloadable copies of the templates
are available from www.bookmarkedhub.com

Further inspiration
To learn more about the authors, their *Menopause Makes*
mission and to see more of their work, visit:

- Websites: www.jenniandkaycreate.co.uk and
  www.menopausemakes.com

- Instagram accounts: @jenniandkaycreate and
  @menopausemakes

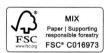

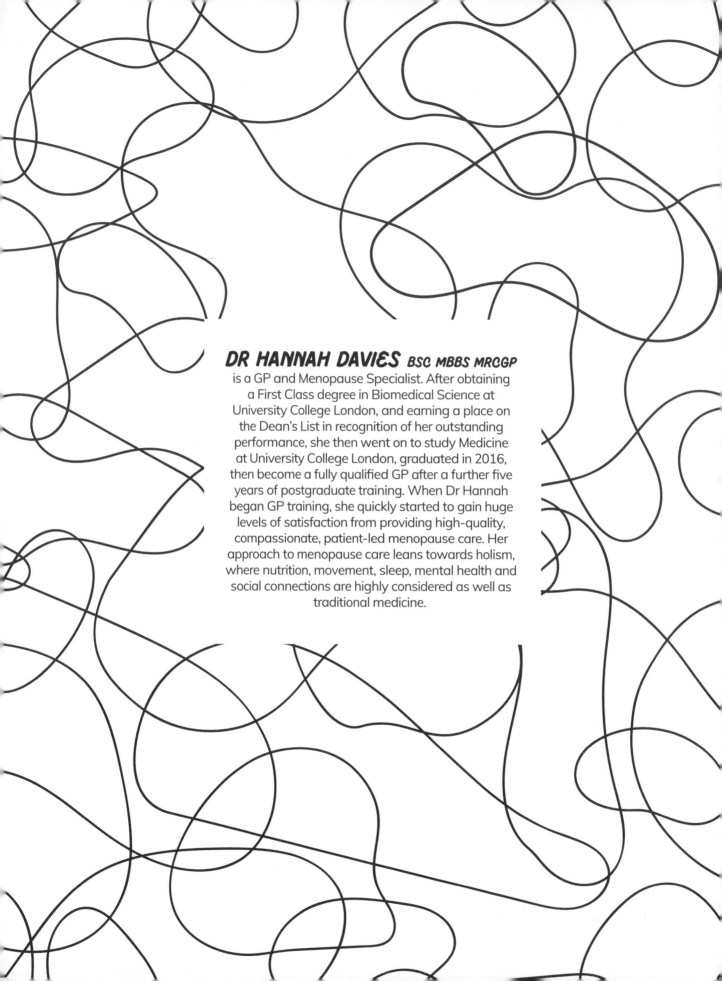

DR HANNAH DAVIES BSc MBBS MRCGP
is a GP and Menopause Specialist. After obtaining
a First Class degree in Biomedical Science at
University College London, and earning a place on
the Dean's List in recognition of her outstanding
performance, she then went on to study Medicine
at University College London, graduated in 2016,
then become a fully qualified GP after a further five
years of postgraduate training. When Dr Hannah
began GP training, she quickly started to gain huge
levels of satisfaction from providing high-quality,
compassionate, patient-led menopause care. Her
approach to menopause care leans towards holism,
where nutrition, movement, sleep, mental health and
social connections are highly considered as well as
traditional medicine.